AMERICAN
ASSOCIATION
of CRITICAL-CARE
NURSES

AACN
Protocols for Practice

Noninvasive Monitoring

Second Edition

Edited by
Suzanne M. Burns
RN, MSN, RRT, ACNP, CCRN,
FAAN, FCCM, FAANP
University of Virginia Health System
Charlottesville, Virginia

JONES AND BARTLETT PUBLISHERS
Sudbury, Massachusetts
BOSTON   TORONTO   LONDON   SINGAPORE

World Headquarters

Jones and Bartlett Publishers
40 Tall Pine Drive
Sudbury, MA 01776
978-443-5000
info@jbpub.com
www.jbpub.com

Jones and Bartlett Publishers Canada
6339 Ormindale Way
Mississauga, Ontario L5V 1J2
CANADA

Jones and Bartlett Publishers International
Barb House, Barb Mews
London W6 7PA
UK

Jones and Bartlett's books and products are available through most bookstores and online booksellers. To contact Jones and Bartlett Publishers directly, call 800-832-0034, fax 978-443-8000, or visit our website, www.jbpub.com.

Substantial discounts on bulk quantities of Jones and Bartlett's publications are available to corporations, professional associations, and other qualified organizations. For details and specific discount information, contact the special sales department at Jones and Bartlett via the above contact information or send an email to specialsales@jbpub.com.

Library of Congress Cataloging-in-Publication Data
Burns, Suzanne M.
    AACN's protocols for practice : noninvasive monitoring / Suzanne Burns.— 2nd ed.
        p. ; cm.
    Includes bibliographical references.
    ISBN 0-7637-3825-5
    1. Hemodynamic monitoring. 2. Diagnosis, Noninvasive.
    [DNLM: 1. Monitoring, Physiologic—instrumentation. 2. Monitoring, Physiologic—methods. 3. Clinical Protocols. 4. Evaluation Studies. 5. Evidence-Based Medicine. WB 142 B967a 2006] I. Title: American Association of Critical-Care Nurses protocols for practice. II. Title: Protocols for practice. III. American Association of Critical-Care Nurses. IV. Title.
    RC670.5.H45B58 2006
    616.1'0754—dc22
                                2005017308

The authors, editor, and publisher have made every effort to provide accurate information. However, they are not responsible for errors, omissions, or for any outcomes related to the use of the contents of this book and take no responsibility for the use of the products described. Treatments and side effects described in this book may not be applicable to all patients; likewise, some patients may require a dose or experience a side effect that is not described herein. The reader should confer with his or her own physician regarding specific treatments and side effects. Drugs and medical devices are discussed that may have limited availability controlled by the Food and Drug Administration (FDA) for use only in a research study or clinical trial. The drug information presented has been derived from reference sources, recently published data, and pharmaceutical research data. Research, clinical practice, and government regulations often change the accepted standard in this field. When consideration is being given to use of any drug in the clinical setting, the health care provider or reader is responsible for determining FDA status of the drug, reading the package insert, reviewing prescribing information for the most up-to-date recommendations on dose, precautions, and contraindications, and determining the appropriate usage for the product. This is especially important in the case of drugs that are new or seldom used.

Production Credits
Acquisitions Editor: Kevin Sullivan
Production Director: Amy Rose
Associate Editor: Amy Sibley
Production Assistant: Alison Meier
Marketing Manager: Emily Ekle
Manufacturing Buyer: Amy Bacus
Composition: Northeast Compositors
Cover Design: Timothy Dziewit
Cover Image: © Photos.com
Printing and Binding: Courier-Stoughton
Cover Printing: Courier-Stoughton

Printed in the United States of America
09 08 07 06 05   10 9 8 7 6 5 4 3 2 1

Contents

iv   **Contents**

About the Protocols

Recognizing that clinical practice must continually evolve to keep up with current science, busy bedside clinicians and advanced practice nurses asked the American Association of Critical-Care Nurses for help in using available research to change acute and critical care practice. They asked for studies to be translated into a format in which findings were demystified and their strength evaluated. They would use this tool to advocate for necessary changes in practice because such changes were based on the latest evidence and because they carried the weight of the association's credibility and influence.

In 1994 the American Association of Critical-Care Nurses began developing research-based practice protocols as one of several responses to this request. AACN's *Protocols for Practice* are designed to provide clinicians at the point of care with the latest patient care research findings in a format that is easy to understand and integrate into clinical practice. The protocols outline the latest thinking on how to best provide care when using technology and in specific patient care situations. Experts in each topic area develop a concise list of recommendations that are appropriate to incorporate into practice routines for patients with a particular situation or device. Recommendations are based on a comprehensive review of the science related to the situation or technology and include only those that are based on research and/or expert consensus positions.

PROTOCOL STRUCTURE

Clinical recommendations represent the core of each protocol. Recommendations are organized in a logical order, usually chronologically, starting with the time before a device is used or an occurrence begins and continuing until after the device is discontinued or the occurrence ends. Recommendations address the following:

Selection of Patients: including indications, contraindications, and special considerations for use, such as age, physiologic status, and intermittent or continuous monitoring. Depending on the device or procedure, a clinical decision-making algorithm may be provided.

Application of Device and Initial Use: where appropriate, important considerations during device or procedure application, such as patient preparation, preapplication calibration, and preparation of application site.

Ongoing Monitoring: important considerations for maintaining the patient during the procedure or for monitoring the device, such as monitoring frequency and clinical factors influencing accuracy and positioning.

Prevention of Complications: key strategies for prevention or early identification of complications, such as infection, skin breakdown, pain, or discomfort.

Quality Control: requirements to maintain accuracy of the device under circumstances of normal use.

Recommendation Level: each recommendation is rated according to the level of information available to support the statement. A scale ranging from I to VI represents progressively stronger levels of scientific basis for the recommendation. Ratings are defined as:

I   Manufacturer's recommendation only.
II Theory-based. No research data to support recommendations. Recommendations from expert consensus groups may exist.
III Laboratory data only. No clinical data to support recommendations.
IV Limited clinical studies to support recommendations.
V   Clinical studies in more than 1 or 2 different populations and situations to support recommendations.
VI Clinical studies in a variety of patient populations and situations to support recommendations.

Along with clinical recommendations, each protocol includes these elements:

- **Case study:** One or more brief case studies describing a common patient care situation related to the protocol topic.
- **General Description:** general description of the device or patient care situation addressed by the protocol.

- **Accuracy:** for medical devices, a general description of the accuracy of the device, including precision and bias, with range of accuracy given when variation exists between models and/or manufacturers.
- **Competency:** specific skill or knowledge verification that is important in determining a nurse's competency.
- **Ethical Considerations:** ethical implications or considerations related to the device or patient care situation.
- **Occupational Hazards:** hazards that may be associated with a device or patient care situation, such as electrical safety or exposure to blood-borne pathogens.
- **Future Research:** suggested areas of future research needed to strengthen the research basis of practice related to the protocol content. This may include key points of research methodology important for clinical studies in this category, such as dependent variables to be measured or confounding variables to be considered.
- **Annotated Bibliography:** summary of important aspects of key studies on the topic.
- **Suggested Readings:** resources for additional information on the protocol topic.

USING THE PROTOCOLS

The protocols are designed to guide care in a variety of acute and critical care settings, including intensive care, progressive care, and medical-surgical units. Selected topics may also be appropriate for long-term and home care. Clinicians should select those elements that apply to their practice setting.

The protocols are not intended to be used as a step-by-step procedure or comprehensive education resource. For this reason, each protocol includes additional information sources. Where available and appropriate, protocols include other essential information such as details about the proper application of devices or patient management algorithms.

Clinicians may consider first using a protocol to assess the topic's current status in their practice. From this baseline assessment, they can evaluate the merits of changing current practice drawing from the protocol's evaluation of evidence that would support a change in practice.

Protocols will be valuable adjuncts in nursing education because they succinctly summarize the state of the science on a specific topic and identify areas for future research. Nursing students are often exposed to wide variation in practice in equally varied clinical settings. Protocols help to identify whether a variation is based on science.

Experienced researchers will find the protocols useful in identifying areas of inquiry. The evidence supporting each action in a protocol is rated according to its level of scientific information. Lower level ratings indicate there is insufficient research to support a strong scientific base. Users with limited expertise in research methods will find that the protocols accurately summarize the research base using a user-friendly, concise approach with minimal jargon. They have been reviewed for scientific merit, readability, and clinical usefulness as of the time of publication.

AACN PRACTICE ALERTS

Recognizing that clinical practice is ever evolving, the American Association of Critical-Care Nurses issues practice alerts as a real-time complement to the protocols. Practice alerts are succinct dynamic directives supported by authoritative evidence to ensure excellence in practice and a safe and humane work environment. The alerts address nursing and multidisciplinary activities of importance to acutely and critically ill patients and environments in order to close the gap between research and practice, provide guidance in changing practice, standardize practice, and identify and inform about advances and new trends in the science. Practice alerts are posted at www.aacn.org.

Acknowledgments

Thanks to the scientific and clinical reviewers who assisted in developing the second edition of these protocols:

- Bedside Cardiac Monitoring—Karen Carlson, Barbara Drew, Gayla Smith

- Respiratory Waveforms Monitoring—Nancy Ames, Jan Headley

- End-Tidal Carbon Dioxide Monitoring—Tom Ahrens, Ronda Bradley, Ginger Braun, Michelle Eichbrecht

- Noninvasive Blood Pressure Monitoring—Ginger Braun, Jan Headley, Nancy Richards

- Pulse Oximetry Monitoring—Tom Ahrens, Mary Lou Sole

Thanks to the AACN national office staff, whose assistance was invaluable to many aspects of the project: Marilyn Herigstad, Justine Medina, and Teresa Wavra.

Special appreciation to Marianne Chulay, who developed and implemented the practice protocols initiative for the American Association of Critical-Care Nurses, and to Barbara Gill MacArthur, executive editor for this series.

Contributors

Suzanne M. Burns, RN, MSN, RRT, ACNP, CCRN,
    FAAN, FCCM, FAANP
Professor of Nursing, Acute and Specialty Care
School of Nursing
Advanced Practice Nurse 2, MICU
University of Virginia Health System
Charlottesville, VA

Karen K. Giuliano, RN, PhD, FAAN
Clinical Research
Philips Medical Systems
Andover, MA

Mary Jo Grap, RN, PhD, ACNP, FAAN
Professor
Virginia Commonwealth University
Adult Health Department
School of Nursing
Richmond, VA

Carol Jacobson, RN, MN
Director
Quality Education Services
Seattle, WA

Robert E. St. John, RN, MSN, RRT
Director, Post-Market Clinical Research
Nellcor/Mallinckrodt—Tyco Healthcare
Pleasanton, CA

Bedside Cardiac Monitoring

Carol Jacobson, RN, MN

CHAPTER ONE

Bedside Cardiac Monitoring

CASE STUDY 1

Mr Perez, a 46-year-old man, was admitted to the emergency department with a wide QRS tachycardia at a rate of 150 beats per minute. His blood pressure was 146/76 mm Hg. He was slightly short of breath but otherwise asymptomatic. The tachycardia did not respond to adenosine or lidocaine, so an elective cardioversion at 50 J was done, and sinus rhythm was restored. Mr Perez was transferred to the telemetry unit for continued monitoring and to await an electrophysiologic study. During the study the next day, ventricular tachycardia was easily induced several times, even after administration of procainamide. Sotalol was started and a follow-up study was scheduled for a few days later when the drug level would be therapeutic. In the meantime, Mr Perez was monitored by telemetry with a 2-lead system, with MCL_1 as the first lead and MCL_6 as the second lead. The day before the follow-up electrophysiologic study, he had another episode of wide QRS tachycardia lasting about 30 seconds that was recorded at the central station in both monitoring leads. The morphology of the tachycardia in MCL_1 and MCL_6 indicated that the rhythm was ventricular tachycardia. A comparison of the findings on the 12-lead electrocardiogram (ECG) of the ventricular tachycardia obtained in the electrophysiologic laboratory showed that the morphology in MCL_1 and MCL_6 was nearly identical to the morphology in V1 and V6 on the 12-lead study, confirming that the spontaneous tachycardia was the same ventricular tachycardia. The recurrence of ventricular tachycardia when Mr Perez was being treated with sotalol indicated that the drug was ineffective in controlling his arrhythmia. The follow-up electrophysiologic study was cancelled, and he was scheduled for placement of an implantable defibrillator. If a less informative lead had been used for monitoring, the nonsustained tachycardia could not have been diagnosed correctly on the basis of information from the monitoring leads, and Mr Perez would have needed the second electrophysiologic study to confirm that sotalol was ineffective in controlling his ventricular tachycardia. The use of optimal bedside monitoring leads for this patient with wide QRS tachycardia eliminated the need for further electrophysiologic testing.

CASE STUDY 2

Ms Bates, a 54-year-old woman, was admitted to the cardiac care unit from the emergency department with an acute myocardial infarction of the anterolateral wall. Her admission ECG showed a 4- to 8-mm ST elevation in leads $V_{1-}V_6$, I, and aVL with reciprocal ST depression in leads II, III, and aVF. The nurses chose lead V1 as the first monitoring lead. Lead aVF was chosen as the second lead for ST-segment monitoring, because aVF was the limb lead that showed the largest ST deviation on the admission ECG taken when Ms Bates was in pain. Thrombolytic therapy with tissue-type plasminogen activator was started within 20 minutes of her arrival in the cardiac care unit. Forty minutes later her ST depression in lead aVF began to resolve, and within 1 hour a 12-lead ECG showed that ST segments had returned almost to baseline in the V leads and in leads I and aVL. During the next 3 hours, her vital signs were stable despite some reperfusion ventricular ectopy, and she was pain free. During hour 4, the ST alarm sounded, and the nurse noted recurrent ST depression in lead aVF. Ms Bates was pain free but slightly hypotensive. A stat 12-lead ECG showed recurrent ST elevation in the anterior leads, and she was returned to the catheterization laboratory for emergency arteriography.

By the time she arrived in the laboratory, she was experiencing 8/10 chest pain. Arteriography showed a reoccluded left anterior descending artery, and percutaneous transluminal coronary angioplasty (PTCA) was performed. The artery was successfully opened, and the ST elevation resolved almost immediately after deflation of the balloon. Ms Bates was returned to the cardiac care unit, where she had an uneventful recovery and no further ST-segment changes during the next 2 days. She was transferred to the telemetry unit, and after 3 days she was discharged from the hospital. The use of ST-segment monitoring in a lead that matched her ischemic fingerprint allowed early detection of her reocclusion, even before the onset of chest pain, leading to immediate intervention to limit myocardial damage.

GENERAL DESCRIPTION

Bedside cardiac monitors used in critical care units, telemetry units, general care floors, operating rooms, postanesthesia recovery units, emergency departments, subacute care units, long-term care facilities, and other areas vary considerably in design, size, special features, and cost. All cardiac monitoring systems allow continuous display of the cardiac rhythm and provide the ability to intermittently make a hard-copy strip recording of the rhythm. The basic components of all cardiac monitoring systems include the following:

- Electrodes that are placed on the patient's chest and detect the electrical impulses generated by cardiac depolarization and repolarization.
- Lead wires attached to the electrodes and a monitoring cable that transmit the electrical impulses to the monitor.
- Amplifier that enlarges the tiny electrical signals generated by the heart.
- Galvanometer that converts the electrical signals to a waveform that can be displayed on a screen.
- Oscilloscope that displays the waveforms of the cardiac cycle. The oscilloscope can be located at the bedside or at a central station on the nursing unit and includes brightness, gain, and sweep-speed controls that allow adjustment of the waveform image for easy viewing.
- Digital heart rate indicator that displays the heart rate in beats per minute.
- Alarm system that activates a sound and/or light alarm if established parameters are violated. A heart rate alarm is standard on all monitoring equipment, but alarms for detection of abnormal beats, runs, and other arrhythmia parameters are available if the system includes computerized arrhythmia detection software.
- Recorder that provides a printed record of the waveforms on a rhythm strip.

In addition to the basic components, many monitoring systems include computer software for detecting arrhythmias that allows more sophisticated monitoring of the rhythm and provides the ability to individualize alarm parameters to individual patients' situations. Some bedside systems now include ST-segment monitoring in addition to arrhythmia detection, and some allow continuous 12-lead ECG monitoring.

ACCURACY

Most currently available bedside monitoring systems display the waveforms of the cardiac rhythm quite accurately. The sensitivity of the ECG for detecting arrhythmia is 100% if the rhythm is being recorded at the time an arrhythmia occurs.[1] Accurate diagnosis of arrhythmias depends on the ability of the observer to analyze the rhythm and use deductive reasoning to determine the mechanism of the arrhythmia.

COMPETENCY

Competency in bedside cardiac monitoring has 4 components:

1. Proper positioning of the electrodes for obtaining specific leads.
2. Optimal lead selection based on the goals of monitoring for each patient's clinical situation.
3. Proper documentation of significant changes in rhythm.
4. Accurate analysis of rhythm strips for correct identification of arrhythmias and recognition of ST-segment deviations.

Staff responsible for ECG monitoring should receive formal orientation and training that is specific to the type of monitoring system used in their clinical area and the goals of monitoring for the patient population served on the unit. Nursing staff should understand specific ECG abnormalities, general electrophysiologic concepts, and be proficient in monitoring skills to work in units where ECG monitoring is a high priority. [2,3,4,5]

Several methods can be used to provide education and document competency. Formal classes and informal bedside teaching on rounds or when giving patients care are ways to provide needed education on bedside monitoring practices. Competency checklists can also be useful tools. Case studies can be used to assess nurses' knowledge about proper selection of leads for particular clinical problems.

Annual skills reviews are a way to assess nurses' knowledge of lead placement. The review can use a written format in which the nurse draws the placement of electrodes on an illustration of a chest and indicates which monitoring wire to attach to each electrode to demonstrate how to obtain a given lead. Actual demonstration of electrode and lead placement can be done on a mannequin at a skills review station.

Periodic audits to assess proper placement of lead V_1 for arrhythmia monitoring and to assess appropriate lead selection at the bedside and central station monitors can help identify educational opportunities and areas where practice changes are needed to ensure current monitoring standards are being met.[4,5]

Any manner of creative teaching or assessment tools can be used to show that nurses can properly identify and document significant changes in rhythm and to assess nurses' monitoring practices.

OCCUPATIONAL HAZARDS

Electrical shock to the nurse and patient can occur if monitoring equipment is faulty or improperly grounded. Severe shock can occur if the cable to the patient is plugged into a direct power source rather than into the proper connection on the monitor.

SUMMARY OF CURRENT RESEARCH

Available research indicates that the best leads for detecting arrhythmia are V_1 and V_6, or MCL_1 and MCL_6 if limited to a 3-wire system. The latest information indicates that when criteria to differentiate wide QRS rhythms are used, V_1 is superior to MCL_1. ST-segment monitoring is a useful tool for detecting myocardial ischemia. The best leads for ST-segment monitoring are those that display the largest ST deviation during an ischemic event (the patient's ST-segment deviation "fingerprint"). The best lead for detecting right coronary artery occlusion is lead III, followed by aVF and then lead II. The best leads for detecting left anterior descending coronary artery occlusion are V_2 and V_3. If limited to limb leads for ST-segment monitoring, the best are those that show maximum ST deviation on the ischemic fingerprint, or leads III and aVF if the fingerprint is not available. If only 2 leads are available for ST-segment monitoring, leads III and V3 are recommended. Continuous 12-lead ST-segment monitoring is superior to any combination of fewer leads for detecting ischemic events.

FUTURE RESEARCH

Additional research in certain areas would be useful. Studies comparing the effectiveness of lead V_1 with lead MCL_1 and leads V_1 or MCL_1 with leads V_6 or MCL_6 in differentiating wide QRS tachycardias in a larger population would add to the excellent initial research by Drew and colleagues[3] in this area.

A study to evaluate the ability of the 12-lead ECG, especially monitoring leads V_1 and/or V_6, to detect loss of capture in the right versus left ventricular pacing leads used for biventricular pacing would be helpful for bedside practitioners. Biventricular pacing has become common for a variety of patients, and evaluating biventricular pacemaker function is a challenge for those providing care.

A study that describes current nursing practice related to the placement of electrodes and the selection of leads and the rationale for the choices being made would further define the problem that exists in this area of practice. Such a study would need to include nurses in all clinical areas in which bedside monitoring is used. A similar study of paramedic practice would be interesting, because much initial information about a patient's heart rhythm and ECG is obtained in the field and transported to the hospital with the patient.

Additional research on the value of continuous 12-lead ECG monitoring in different populations of patients, including those in the operating room, from a nursing and a cost-control perspective would be valuable. Most studies of this type have been directed at the value of intraoperative or postoperative 12-lead ECG monitoring in detecting silent ischemia and in enabling healthcare providers to intervene earlier in surgical patients with coronary artery disease, but does it really make a difference in patients' outcome or lead to earlier discharge? Does continuous 12-lead ECG monitoring for ischemia have any value in directing nursing interventions? Can ST-segment monitoring be used in a way similar to SVO_2 monitoring as an indicator of a patient's response to nursing or other interventions?

Studies are also needed that examine the methods, efficacy, and cost of using cardiac monitoring in general medical-surgical units in patients treated with beta-blockers after noncardiac surgery. Recent studies suggest that the administration of beta-blockers before, during, and after noncardiac surgery reduces the risk of adverse cardiac events and improves survival in high-risk patients.[6] Adoption of this practice creates a need for hospitals to decide where (eg, critical care, telemetry, or general medical-surgical unit) and how (eg, hard-wire, telemetry, central stations on the unit, or remote monitoring) to monitor these patients, and what type of training to provide for nurses who are not used to cardiac monitoring.

REFERENCES

1. Fisch C. Electrocardiogram and mechanisms of arrhythmias. In: Podrid PJ, Kowrey PR, eds. *Cardiac Arrhythmia: Mechanisms, Diagnosis, and Management.* Baltimore, Md: Williams & Wilkins; 1995:211.
2. Drew BJ, Krucoff MW. Multilead ST-segment monitoring in patients with acute coronary syndromes: a consensus statement for healthcare professionals. *Am J Crit Care.* 1999; 8:372.

3. Drew BJ, Scheinman MM. Value of electrocardiographic leads MCL$_1$, MCL$_6$, and other selected leads in the diagnosis of wide QRS complex tachycardia. *J Am Coll Cardiol.* 1991;18:1025–1033.
4. American Association of Critical-Care Nurses. *Practice Alert: Dysrhythmia Monitoring.* AACN, Aliso Viejo, Calif. Available at: http://www.accn.org/PracticeAlerts. Accessed July 7, 2005.
5. American Association of Critical-Care Nurses. *Practice Alert: ST-Segment Monitoring.* AACN, Aliso Viejo, Calif. Available at: http://www.accn.org/PracticeAlerts. Accessed July 7, 2005.
6. Auerbach AD, Goldman L. Beta-blockers and reduction of cardiac events in noncardiac surgery. *JAMA.* 2002;287:1435.

CLINICAL RECOMMENDATIONS

The rating scales for the Level of Recommendation column range from I to VI, with levels indicated as follows: I, manufacturer's recommendation only; II, theory based, no research data to support recommendations; recommendations from expert consensus group may exist; III, laboratory data only, no clinical data to support recommendations; IV, limited clinical studies to support recommendations; V, clinical studies in more than 1 or 2 different populations and situations to support recommendations; VI, clinical studies in a variety of patient populations and situations to support recommendations.

Period of Use	Recommendation	Rationale for Recommendation	Level of Recommendation	Supporting References	Comments
Selection of Patients	Bedside cardiac monitoring should be used under the following circumstances:				
	CARDIAC ARRHYTHMIA MONITORING *Class I (indicated in most, if not all, patients in this group)*		II: Theory based, no research data to support recommendations; expert consensus document does exist	See Reference 3	Randomized clinical trials in bedside cardiac monitoring are almost nonexistent. The purpose of the consensus document (see Reference 3) is to provide "best practices" for hospital ECG monitoring in the absence of research in the area.
	• Patients who have been resuscitated from cardiac arrest	Patients resuscitated from cardiac arrest are at high risk for recurrence of that event.			
	• Patients in the early phase of acute coronary syndromes (ST elevation or non-ST elevation myocardial infarction [MI]; unstable angina/"rule out" MI)	Arrhythmias are the most common complication of ischemic heart disease and acute coronary syndrome (ACS).			
	• Patients with unstable coronary syndromes and newly diagnosed high risk coronary lesions	Reperfusion arrhythmias are common during and after administration of thrombolytic agents for ACS.			
	• Adults and children who have undergone cardiac surgery	Detection of potentially lethal and other significant arrhythmias allows early treatment to avoid sudden death and other complications in patients with ACS and following cardiac surgery.			
	• Patients who have undergone non-urgent percutaneous coronary intervention who have complications	Monitoring is indicated for patients who have complications in the cath lab (eg, vessel dissection, no reflow, serious arrhythmias) or who have suboptimal interventional outcomes.			

Period of Use	Recommendation	Rationale for Recommendation	Level of Recommendation	Supporting References	Comments
Selection of Patients (*cont.*)	• Patients who have undergone implantation of an automatic defibrillator lead or a pacemaker lead and who are considered pacemaker dependent	Loss of capture in a pacemaker-dependent patient can lead to asystole and death and must be immediately recognized a corrected.			
	• Patients with a temporary pacemaker or transcutaneous pacing pads	Loss of capture and sensing in a temporary or permanent pacemaker can lead to hemodynamic instability requiring immediate treatment.			
	• Patients with AV block	Type II second-degree block, high-grade block, and third-degree block can result in symptomatic bradycardia and hemodynamic instability requiring immediate treatment.			
	• Patients with arrhythmias complicating Wolff- Parkinson-White Syndrome (WPW) with rapid anterograde conduction over an accessory pathway	Anterograde conduction over an accessory pathway can lead to rapid ventricular rates and sudden cardiac death.			
	• Patients with long QT syndrome and associated ventricular arrhythmias	Torsades de Pointes is a life-threatening ventricular tachyarrhythmia associated with a prolonged QT interval that can result in sudden cardiac death. Episodes of Torsades are often preceded by pauses or polymorphic ventricular beats that can be recognized through cardiac monitoring. Torsades can degenerate into ventricular fibrillation, which requires immediate recognition and treatment.			
	• Patients receiving intra-aortic balloon counterpulsation	Many arrhythmias make tracking by the IABP difficult and lead to ineffective pumping			
	• Patients with acute heart failure/pulmonary edema	Several arrhythmias can contribute to or be a cause of acute heart failure. Heart failure is a risk factor for development of many arrhythmias.			

Period of Use	Recommendation	Rationale for Recommendation	Level of Recommendation	Supporting References	Comments
Selection of Patients (*cont.*)	• Patients with indications for intensive care	ECG monitoring is recommended for patients with major trauma, acute respiratory failure, sepsis, shock, acute pulmonary embolus, major surgery, renal failure with electrolyte abnormalities, drug overdose.			
	• Patients undergoing diagnostic or therapeutic procedures requiring conscious sedation or anesthesia				
	• Patients with any other hemodynamically unstable arrhythmia				
	Class II (ECG monitoring may be of benefit in some patients but is not considered essential for all)		II: Theory based, no research data to support recommendations; expert consensus document does exist	See Reference 3	
	• Patients post-acute MI (defined as 24–48 hours after hospital admission)	Patients with prior hypertension, chronic obstructive pulmonary disease, prior MI, ST-segment changes at presentation, higher Killip Class, and lower initial systolic blood pressure may be at higher risk for in-hospital sustained ventricular arrhythmias.			
	• Patients with chest pain syndromes	Patients who present with chest pain but do not have diagnostic ECG findings or elevated biomarkers may benefit from telemetry monitoring if they also have: low systolic blood pressure (< 110 mm Hg), pulmonary rales above the bases bilaterally, or a history of unstable ischemic heart disease.			
	• Patients who have undergone uncomplicated, nonurgent percutaneous coronary interventions (ie, not for acute MI)	Monitoring for 6–8 hours after the procedure is recommended if the patient received a stent. Patients who undergo coronary angioplasty without stenting may benefit from monitoring for 12–24 hours.			

Period of Use	Recommendation	Rationale for Recommendation	Level of Recommendation	Supporting References	Comments
Selection of Patients (*cont.*)	• Patients who are being started on an antiarrhythmic drug or who require adjustment of drugs for rate control with chronic atrial tachyarrhythmias	Benefits of monitoring include assessment of efficacy of drug therapy and detection of the following potential adverse effects of antiarrhythmic drug therapy: prolonging QT interval, bradycardia, AV block, proarrhythmia, hemodynamic deterioration due to negative inotropic effects of some antiarrhythmics.			
	• Patients who have undergone implantation of a pacemaker lead and who are not pacemaker dependent	Monitoring recommended for 12–24 hours to evaluate proper pacemaker function and programming.			
	• Patients who have undergone uncomplicated ablation of an arrhythmia	Monitoring recommended for 12–24 hours in patients who have had prolonged rapid heart rates from incessant tachycardia, patients who have been in chronic atrial fibrillation and have undergone AV node ablation with pacemaker implant, and patients with significant organic heart disease who undergo ventricular tachycardia ablation.			
	• Patients who have undergone routine coronary angiography	Monitoring is beneficial in detecting vaso-vagal reactions during and after sheath removal following femoral artery access.			
	• Patients with subacute heart failure	Monitoring may be beneficial in these patients while medications and/or device therapy are being manipulated.			
	• Patients who are being evaluated for syncope	Monitoring recommended for 24–48 hours in patients in whom there is suspicion about an arrhythmic cause of syncope or who have conduction system disease, non-sustained ventricular tachycardia, or possible pacemaker malfunction.			
	• Patients with "Do not resuscitate" orders who have arrhythmias causing discomfort	Goal of monitoring is to assist in titrating antiarrhythmic drugs for optimum rate control as part of "comfort" care in patients who experience palpitations, shortness of breath, or anxiety.			

Period of Use	Recommendation	Rationale for Recommendation	Level of Recommendation	Supporting References	Comments
Selection of Patients (*cont.*)	ST SEGMENT ISCHEMIA MONITORING				
	Class I (ST-segment monitoring is indicated in most, if not all, patients in this group): • Patients in the early phase of acute coronary syndromes (ST elevation or no-ST elevation MI; unstable angina/"Rule out" MI)	Patients with ACS are the highest priority for ST-segment monitoring. Potential benefits of monitoring in these patients include the ability to assess patency of the culprit artery after thrombolytic therapy; detect reocclusion after percutaneous coronary interventions (PCI); detect ongoing, recurrent, or transient ischemia; detect infarct expansion.	II: Theory based, no research data to support recommendations; expert consensus document does exist	See Reference 3	
	• Patients who present to the emergency department with chest pain or anginal equivalent symptoms	Patients with acute MI often have an initial ECG that is non-diagnostic for acute ischemia. Initiation of ST-segment monitoring in the emergency department can facilitate recognition of acute MI in these patients as well as prevent patients from being discharged inappropriately.			
	• Patients who have undergone non-urgent percutaneous coronary intervention who have suboptimal angiographic results	Patients who have complications in the cath lab (eg, vessel dissection or thrombosis), or who have suboptimal interventional results may be at higher risk for abrupt reocclusion.			
	• Patients with possible variant angina due to coronary vasospasm	Potential benefits of ST-segment monitoring in these patients include the ability to confirm the diagnosis by detecting transient ST-segment elevation, predict the culprit artery, assess risk for malignant ventricular arrhythmias during vasospasm, and assess efficacy of therapy with calcium channel blockers.			
	Class II (ST-segment monitoring may be of benefit in some patients but is not considered essential for all): • Patients with post-acute MI (after 24–48 hours)	ST-segment monitoring should continue in patients who have had recurrent chest pain or anginal symptoms or who have had a second rise of cardiac enzymes indicating infarct extension.	II: Theory based, no research data to support recommendations; expert consensus document does exist		

Period of Use	Recommendation	Rationale for Recommendation	Level of Recommendation	Supporting References	Comments
Selection of Patients (*cont.*)	• Patients who have undergone non-urgent, uncomplicated percutaneous coronary intervention	Many patients experience chest pain following PCI that may or may not be related to ischemia. ST-segment monitoring can assist in the evaluation of post-procedure chest pain.			
	• Patients at high risk for ischemia after cardiac or noncardiac surgery	In cardiac surgery patients, ST-segment monitoring can assist in distinguishing incisional pain from ischemic chest pain, assess graft patency, detect reocclusion, and determine whether post-operative cardiac arrhythmias or heart failure have an ischemic basis. In noncardiac surgical patients, ST-segment monitoring can detect perioperative ischemia in high risk patients (eg, elderly, patients having emergent major operations, aortic and other major vascular surgery, prolonged surgical procedures).			
	• Pediatric patients at risk of ischemia or infarction due to congenital or acquired conditions				
	Class III (ST-segment monitoring is not recommended because of the increased incidence of false ST alarms in these situations):				
	• Patients with left bundle-branch block	LBBB causes marked ST T-wave deviation that varies with heart rate and triggers frequent false ST alarms			
	• Patients with ventricular-paced rhythms	This same rationale applies to patients with ventricular pacemakers.			
	• Patients with other confounding arrhythmias that obscure the ST segment (ie, course atrial fibrillation or flutter, intermittent accelerated ventricular rhythm)	These rhythms create fluctuations in the ST segment that triggers frequent false ST alarms.			
	• Patients who are agitated	Agitation creates noisy signals that cause frequent false ST alarms.			

Period of Use	Recommendation	Rationale for Recommendation	Level of Recommendation	Supporting References	Comments
Application of Device and Initial Monitoring	**SKIN PREPARATION:** Prepare the patient's skin as follows: 1. Shave hair from the electrode site if necessary. 2. Wash the skin with soap and water and dry it thoroughly. 3. Clean the skin at the electrode site with alcohol. 4. With a dry washcloth, a gauze pad, or the abrasive pad on the electrode, gently abrade the skin where the electrode gel pad will be placed. 5. If the patient is diaphoretic, apply tincture of benzoin to the skin where the electrode adhesive will be placed. Do not apply benzoin to the center area where the electrode gel will contact the skin.	Reducing skin resistance improves the quality of the signal and decreases the number of artifacts.	IV: Limited clinical studies to support recommendations	See Annotated Bibliography: 2, 3 See Reference 3 See Other References: 1	
	ELECTRODE PREPARATION: Prepare the electrodes as follows: 1. Connect the electrodes to the lead wires. 2. Peel the paper from the adhesive on each electrode, and attach the electrode to the appropriate site by pressing the adhesive onto the patient's skin. Avoid pressing on the gel pad. 3. Make a stress-loop and secure the lead wires to the patient's chest if the patient is active. 4. Secure the cable to the patient's gown or place the telemetry transmitter in a carrying pouch or pocket.	Connecting the wires to the electrodes first avoids pressure on the gel part of the electrode and prevents spreading gel onto the adhesive surface. This technique is also more comfortable for the patient.		See Other References: 2	

Period of Use	Recommendation	Rationale for Recommendation	Level of Recommendation	Supporting References	Comments
Application of Device and Initial Monitoring (*cont.*)	ARRYTHMIA MONITORING Place the electrodes and select the leads as follows: *Three-Wire System, Lead MCL_1 and MCL_6* 1. Attach the right arm (RA) wire to an electrode on the patient's left shoulder. 2. Attach the left arm (LA) wire to an electrode at the V_1 position (fourth intercostals space at right sternal border). 3. Attach the left leg (LL) wire to an electrode at the V_6 position (fifth intercostals space at left midaxillary line). 4. With lead wires in this position, select lead I on the bedside monitoring to get MCL_1. Select lead II on the bedside monitor to get MCL_6.	Proper positioning of the electrodes and correct attachment of the lead wires are extremely important. MCL_1 is the best lead for bedside arrhythmia monitoring if a 3-lead system must be used. MCL_6 is the second best lead if placing an electrode in the V_1 position is impossible because of dressings.	IV: Limited clinical studies to support recommendations	See Annotated Bibliography: 4–6, 9 See Other References: 3–5, 11	Refer to Figure 1 Research indicates that a true unipolar V1 lead obtained with a five-lead system is superior to the modified bipolar MCL_1 lead in differentiating wide QRS tachycardias.
	Five-Wire System 1. Attach the arm electrodes to the patient's shoulders (front, top, or back) close to where the arms join the torso: • RA wire to right shoulder • LA wire to left shoulder 2. Attach the leg electrodes low on the thorax at the level of the lowest rib, on the abdomen, or on the hips: • RL to right side • LL to left side	Limb electrodes need to be attached close to where the limbs join the torso to provide the most accurate reading of cardiac activity. Arm electrodes placed medially under the clavicle, or leg electrodes placed too high on the rib cage alter the point of view of the leads and result in inaccurate recording.	IV: Limited clinical studies to support recommendations	See Annotated Bibliography: 4–6, 9 See Other References: 3–5	Refer to Figure 2

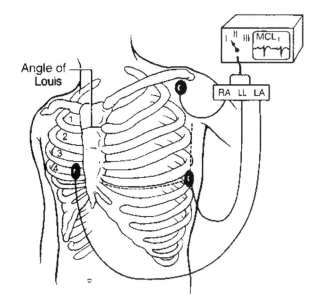

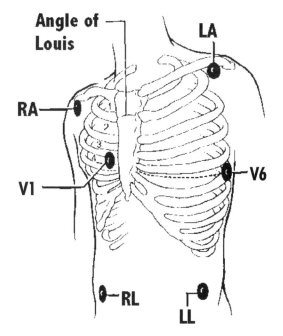

Figure 1.1: Electrode palcement for a three-wire system. Drew JB. Bedside electrocardiogram monitoring. *AACN Clin Issues.* 1993;4:25–33. (Reprinted with permission.)

Figure 1.2: Electrode placement for a three-wire system. Drew BJ. Bedside electrocardiogram monitoring. *AACN Clin Issues.* 1993;4:25–33. (Reprinted with permission.)

Period of Use	Recommendation	Rationale for Recommendation	Level of Recommendation	Supporting References	Comments
Application of Device and Initial Monitoring (*cont.*)	3. Place the chest electrode at the V_1 position (fourth intercostal space at the right sternal border) to record V_1 or at the V_6 position (fifth intercostal space, left midaxillary line) to record V_6. 4. Select V on the bedside monitor to record V_1 or V_6, depending on where the chest electrode is placed, or select desired frontal plane lead to record leads I, II, III, aVR, aVL, and aVF. **ST-SEGMENT MONITORIN** Choose the monitoring leads according to the following guidelines:	V_1 is the lead of choice for bedside monitoring with a 5-lead system. V_6 is the second best choice if placing an electrode in the V_1 position is impossible because of dressings. If the bedside monitor offers a choice between a V lead or an MCL lead, choose the V lead, because the true V_1 is more accurate than MCL_1 in some wide QRS tachycardias.			

Period of Use	Recommendation	Rationale for Recommendation	Level of Recommendation	Supporting References	Comments
Application of Device and Initial Monitoring (*cont.*)	*If Continuous 12-Lead ST-Segment Monitoring Is Available* 1. Monitor all 12 leads and set alarms to sound if ST segment changes 1 to 2 mm in any lead. ST-segment monitors have default alarms that can be used, but the alarms should be individualized for each patient whenever possible.	Continuous 12-lead ST-segment monitoring is the most reliable noninvasive way to detect silent ischemia and coronary artery reocclusion in patients with ACS and after thrombolytic therapy or PCI. 12-Lead monitoring allows the use of all limb leads and all V leads simultaneously, eliminating the need to rely on limb leads exclusively for ST-segment monitoring and avoiding the need to choose the *best* leads for the patient's clinical situation. Simultaneous V leads provide the 2 best leads (V_1 and V_6) for monitoring arrhythmia and the best leads (V_2 and V_3) for monitoring ST segments in anterior myocardial infarction and interventions in the left anterior descending artery.	IV: Limited clinical studies to support recommendations	See Annotated Bibliography: 10–12, 14–17 See Other References: 6–9	
	Five-Wire, Multi-lead Monitoring System 1. Position the limb electrodes for a 5-lead system (see Figure 2).		IV: Limited clinical studies to support recommendations	See Annotated Bibliography: 1, 10–12, 14	
	2. Use the chest electrode to obtain lead V_1 (or V_6 if V_1 cannot be used) for monitoring arrhythmia in all multi-lead combinations if the patient is at risk for developing significant arrhythmias.	Detection of arrhythmia remains the primary goal of bedside monitoring in most patients with coronary disease, and V_1 is the best lead for this purpose.			
	3. Use the chest electrode for ST-segment monitoring in lead V_3 if the patient has acute coronary syndrome.	If the patient has acute coronary syndrome, ST-segment monitoring may be more important than arrhythmia monitoring. Lead V_2 or V_3 are the best leads for detecting left anterior coronary artery occlusion.		See Annotated Bibliography: 1, 11, 16	

Period of Use	Recommendation	Rationale for Recommendation	Level of Recommendation	Supporting References	Comments
Application of Device and Initial Monitoring (*cont.*)	*If 2 Monitoring Leads Are Available* 1. If using lead V_1 for arrhythmia monitoring, choose the second lead on the basis of the patient's *ischemic fingerprint* obtained during chest pain or during balloon inflation during PCI. Use the limb lead with the largest ST-segment deviation (elevation or depression).	Most current bedside monitors allow recording of only one V lead at a time. If V_1 is used to detect arrhythmia, the second lead would be limited to a limb lead.	IV: Limited clinical studies to support recommendations	See Annotated Bibliography: 1, 9–12, 16	
	2. If no ischemic fingerprint is available, choose either lead III or lead aVF for the second monitoring lead (whichever has the largest R wave)	Leads III and aVF are the most valuable limb leads for detecting ischemia related to occlusion in all 3 major coronary arteries.			
	If 3 Monitoring Leads Are Available 1. Use V_1 for arrhythmia monitoring and use the patient's ischemic fingerprint to choose the second and third leads for ST-segment monitoring. If no ischemic fingerprint is available, the combination of V_1, lead I, and lead aVF offer several advantages.	This combination provides the best lead (V_1) for monitoring arrhythmia, anterior and lateral leads (V_1 and I), and an inferior lead (aVF) for ST-segment monitoring. It also provides the ability to quickly determine the electrical axis by using leads I and aVF.	IV: Limited clinical studies to support recommendations	See Annotated Bibliography: 12	
	2. If more than 1 V lead is available, use V_1 for arrhythmia monitoring, V_3 and lead III for ST-segment monitoring.	V_3 is one of the best leads for anterior wall ST-segment monitoring, and lead III is best for inferior wall ST-segment monitoring.		See Annotated Bibliography: 10, 11, 16	
	ADJUSTING THE MONITOR AND SETTING ALARMS Adjust the monitor and set the alarms as follows:				

Period of Use	Recommendation	Rationale for Recommendation	Level of Recommendation	Supporting References	Comments
Application of Device and Initial Monitoring (*cont.*)	1. Adjust the gain on the monitor so the amplitude of QRS is large enough to be detected by the heart rate counter but not so large that the QRS complex is cut off at the top or bottom. Be sure the monitor is not double-counting T waves.	The accuracy of the alarm system depends on an adequate signal for the heart rate counter to detect. The heart rate meter counts the tallest deflections seen. If the T wave is nearly equal to the QRS complex in size, double-counting can occur, resulting in alarms because of falsely high heart rates.	II: Theory based, no research data to support recommendations		
	2. Set the heart rate alarm limits on the basis of the patient's clinical situation and current heart rate. Most monitoring systems have default alarms that adjust the high- and low-rate limits on the basis of the learned heart rate.		I: Manufacturer's recommendation only		
	3. Set the alarm limits on other parameters if using a computerized arrhythmia monitoring system. Each system has its own default alarms that can be individualized as needed.				Most computerized systems for monitoring arrhythmia have default alarms for each arrhythmia parameter. It is always best to individualize alarms for each patient, especially if the defaults are inappropriate for the clinical situation.
Ongoing Monitoring	Observe the skin at the electrode sites daily. Remove the electrodes, wash the skin, and apply lotion or other skin care products if irritation is severe. Reposition the electrodes if signs of skin irritation are present, maintaining proper positioning of the electrodes whenever possible.	Adhesive or gel on the electrode can cause skin irritation and discomfort. It may be necessary to monitor V_6 if the V_1 site is irritated.	I: Manufacturer's recommendation only	See Annotated Bibliography: 13	
	Replace the electrodes every 48 hours.	Replacing the electrodes prevents drying of the gel.			
	If one electrode requires replacement, replace all the electrodes at the same time.	Electrode resistance changes as the gel dries, so changing all electrodes at once prevents differences in resistance between electrodes.			

Period of Use	Recommendation	Rationale for Recommendation	Level of Recommendation	Supporting References	Comments
Ongoing Monitoring (*cont.*) **Device Removal** **Prevention of Complications**	Check placement of the electrodes and selection of the leads every shift to verify proper monitoring technique.	Verification of accurate positioning of the electrodes and proper lead selection based on the patient's clinical situation provides optimal monitoring for each patient and quality control among the nursing staff.			
	Document rhythm strip on admission, every shift, and with significant change in rhythm. Document heart rate, PR interval, and QRS width on rhythm strip at least once per shift and with every significant change in rhythm.				
	Document the monitoring lead on every rhythm strip.	Accurate interpretation of many arrhythmias depends on knowing which lead is being monitored.			Many clues to rhythm identification are lead specific and can only be used when the correct lead is examined.
	To remove the monitoring system, first turn off the bedside monitor. Then carefully peel the electrode from the skin. Wash the skin and apply lotion or other skin care product if irritation is present.	Turning off the monitoring system first avoids triggering the alarm system.	I: Manufacturer's recommendation only		
	Steps to prevent complications include the following: • Observe the skin and provide skin care as recommended to prevent skin irritation. • Make sure all electrical equipment is properly grounded. • Report persistent electrical interference on the monitor to the engineering staff.	If proper skin preparation and securing lead wires does not eliminate electrical interference, the cause could be interference from an external source or faulty equipment grounding and may be an electrical hazard to the patient.	II: Theory based, no research data to support	See Other References: 1, 10	

Period of Use	Recommendation	Rationale for Recommendation	Level of Recommendation	Supporting References	Comments
Quality Control Issues	Four areas of quality control and competency verification apply to ECG monitoring:		II: Theory based, no research data to support recommendations; consensus document does exist.	See Annotated Bibliography: 7, 8, 16, 17	
	1. Proper electrode positioning for obtaining specific leads	Accurate recording of cardiac electrical activity depends on proper skin preparation and proper placement of the electrodes that are doing the recording. Even minor errors in position (especially in V_1) can alter the recording and invalidate many of the ECG clues used to identify arrhythmias, especially wide QRS rhythms.			
	2. Optimal lead selection based on the goals of monitoring for each patient's clinical situation	The goals of monitoring for each patient should determine lead selection, rather than standard unit policy or manufacturers' recommendations.			
		Consider whether the patient is at risk for significant arrhythmias, especially wide QRS rhythms, and choose a lead that gives the most information: V_1 or V6. Many arrhythmias are transient, and once they have occurred, it is too late to go back and pick a better monitoring lead.			
		Choose ST-segment monitoring leads according to the patient's clinical presentation; i.e., use leads recommended for detection of ischemia in the artery involved in the patient's clinical situation.			
	3. Proper documentation of significant changes in rhythm	Placing a rhythm strip in the chart for each significant change in rhythm is essential.			
		Documenting many rhythm changes, especially tachycardias (narrow or wide QRS) with a full 12-lead ECG is helpful in determining the mechanism of the arrhythmia.			
		Indicating the monitoring lead on each rhythm strip is essential in analyzing many arrhythmias, especially wide QRS rhythms. Because lead selection may vary with the clinical situation from shift to shift, the lead should be noted on every strip.			

Period of Use	Recommendation	Rationale for Recommendation	Level of Recommendation	Supporting References	Comments
Quality Control Issues (*cont.*)	4. Knowledge and skills in cardiac monitoring, arrhythmia identification, and in recognition of ST-segment deviations.	Nursing staff should be knowledgeable in general electrophysiology concepts, specific ECG abnormalities, and be proficient in monitoring skills to work in units where ECG monitoring is a high priority.		See Annotated Bibliography: 16, 17	

ANNOTATED BIBLIOGRAPHY

1. Aldrich HR, Hindman NB, Hinohara T, et al. Identification of the optimal electrocardiographic leads for detecting acute epicardial injury in acute myocardial infarction. *Am J Cardiol*. 1987;59:20–23.

Study Sample

The sample population consisted of 148 patients with acute myocardial infarction verified by ECG findings and enzyme tests. The study included patients with inferior (n = 80) and anterior (n = 68) myocardial infarction.

Comparison Studied

The study determined the amount of ST-segment deviation (either elevation or depression) in each of the 12 leads (except aVR) present with inferior and anterior myocardial infarction.

Study Procedures

The study population was selected from patients admitted during 1965 to 1981 who met several inclusion criteria for acute myocardial infarction. ST-segment deviation was measured, and the location of the infarction was determined on the basis of the lead with the maximum ST deviation.

Key Results

In patients with inferior infarctions, lead III was the most frequent location for ST elevation (94%) and the most common lead with maximal ST deviation. In patients with anterior infarctions, lead V_2 had the highest frequency of ST elevation (99%), and leads V_2 and V_3 were the most common sites of maximal ST elevation.

Study Strengths and Weaknesses

The study examined only the initial ECGs of patients with acute myocardial infarction. Serial ECGs were not examined. Studies of patients receiving thrombolytic therapy are needed to determine if ECG leads can be used to detect coronary artery reocclusion. The authors' recommendations for best monitoring leads do not consider the goal of arrhythmia detection. Their recommendations are only for monitoring ischemia.

Clinical Implications

The authors suggest that monitoring in leads V_2 and III is superior to monitoring in leads V_1 and II for detecting ST-segment deviation in acute myocardial infarction.

2. Medina V, Clochesy JM, Omery A. Comparison of electrode site preparation techniques. *Heart Lung*. 1989;18:456–460.

Study Sample

Healthy adults (n = 60).

Comparison Studied

Three skin preparation techniques were compared for their ability to decrease skin resistance and decrease the offset potential between 2 electrodes. The first technique, SPT-A, consisted of five strokes with an alcohol pad. The second, SPT-B, consisted of 5 strokes with an alcohol pad and 1 stroke with One Step Skin Prep (an abrasive product). The third, SPT-C, consisted of 5 strokes with an alcohol pad and 5 strokes with an ECG Prep Pad (an abrasive product).

Study Procedures

Subjects were randomly assigned to 2 treatment groups or a control group (20 subjects in each). Offset potential between electrode pairs was measured with a digital multimeter.

Key Results

Both SPT-B and SPT-C, which were abrasive techniques, reduced offset potential. Results with SPT-A were mixed.

Study Strengths and Weaknesses

The study had a small sample size. Subjects were healthy adults, so factors affecting patients in critical care units, such as effects of certain disease states on skin or effects of excessive perspiration, were not studied.

Clinical Implications

Artifacts associated with the interface between ECG electrodes and the skin can be minimized by using abrasive skin preparation techniques.

3. Clochesy JM, Cifani L, Howe K. Electrode site preparation techniques: a follow-up study. *Heart Lung*. 1991;20:27–30.

Study Sample

Healthy adults (n = 120).

Comparison Studied

Four different skin preparation techniques were compared for their ability to decrease skin resistance and decrease the offset potential between 2 electrodes. The first technique, SPT 1, consisted of 5 strokes with alcohol pad and 1 stroke with One Step Skin Prep. The second, SPT 2, consisted of 5 strokes with an alcohol pad and 5 strokes with an ECG Prep Pad. The third, SPT 3, consisted of 5 strokes with an alcohol pad and 1 stroke with an ECG Prep Pad. The fourth, SPT 4, consisted of 5 strokes with an alcohol pad.

Study Procedures

Subjects were randomly assigned to 1 of 3 treatment groups or the control group (30 subjects in each group). Offset potential between electrode pairs was measured with 2 different meters.

Key Results

Statistically significant decreases in offset potential were found in the SPT 1 and SPT 3 groups.

Study Strengths and Weaknesses

This study was a replication of the previous study by Medina, Clochesy, and Omery (reference 2 in this bibliography). Similar results were obtained, confirming that artifacts caused by the interface between ECG electrodes and the skin can be significantly reduced by mild skin abrasion. Subjects were healthy adults, so factors affecting patients in critical care units, such as effects of certain disease states on skin or effects of excessive perspiration, were not studied.

Clinical Implications

Artifacts associated with the interface between ECG electrodes and the skin can be minimized by using abrasive skin preparation techniques.

4. Drew BJ, Scheinman MM, Dracup K. MCL_1 and MCL_6 compared to V_1 and V_6 in distinguishing aberrant supraventricular from ventricular ectopic beats. *Pacing Clin Electrophysiol.* 1991;14:1375–1383.

Study Sample

Isolated wide QRS beats (n = 81) were recorded from 46 adults in a cardiac electrophysiology laboratory.

Comparison Studied

The similarity in QRS was compared between leads V_1 and MCL_1 and between leads V_6 and MCL_6 to determine the accuracy of the modified leads commonly used in bedside monitoring as substitutes for true V leads. An additional goal of this study was to determine if the measurement from onset of QRS to tallest peak or nadir of QRS is a useful criterion for differentiating aberration from ventricular ectopy.

Study Procedures

Information from leads MCL_1, MCL_6, V_1, and V_6 and intracardiac leads was recorded in all patients. The electrode wires for leads MCL_1 and V_1 were soldered together, as were the ones for leads MCL_6 and V_6, because the same spot on the chest is required to record more than 1 lead. Each of the 81 abnormal beats was examined in leads V_1, V_6, MCL_1, and MCL_6 for evidence of well-established crite-

ria for QRS morphology used to differentiate aberrancy from ventricular ectopy. In addition, measurements from onset of QRS to tallest peak or to nadir of QRS were made to determine the usefulness of the new criterion. Two independent observers evaluated the complexes, and their diagnosis, based on established criteria for QRS morphology, was compared with the true diagnosis as determined by using intracardiac leads.

Key Results

Bipolar precordial leads MCL_1 and MCL_6 were valid substitutes for unipolar leads V_1 and V_6. The MCL_1 and V_1 leads were superior to the MCL_6 and V_6 leads for correct diagnosis of the origin of wide QRS complexes. The QRS morphology in leads MCL_1 and V_1 was clearly different in 9% of wide QRS beats (this did not affect diagnostic accuracy). The new criterion, measuring from onset of QRS to tallest peak or nadir in V_6 or MCL_6, showed that a measurement of 50 milliseconds or less favors a supraventricular origin, whereas a measurement of 70 milliseconds or more favors a ventricular origin. The same measurement in lead V_1 or lead MCL_1 was helpful in complexes with the morphology of left bundle-branch block but not in those with the morphology of right bundle-branch block. When the new criterion was used with lead V_6 or lead MCL_6, there was no difference between the 4 leads for diagnosis of wide QRS complexes.

Study Strengths and Weaknesses

This study reconfirmed previously published criteria for differentiating wide QRS complexes with the morphology of both right and left bundle-branch blocks. This study validated the use of leads MCL_1 and MCL_6 as substitutes for leads V_1 and V_6 for bedside monitoring. The study proposes the use of the new criterion with lead V_6 or lead MCL_6 as an additional aid in differentiating wide QRS complexes. The sample size of 81 beats was fairly small. A larger sample size would be helpful, especially with wide QRS beats that differ between leads V_1 and MCL_1.

Clinical Implications

Using lead MCL_1 or lead MCL_6 is recommended for monitoring for arrhythmias when lead V_1 or lead V_6 cannot be used, as is the case with a 3-wire system. Use of established criteria for differentiating the origin of wide QRS complex beats is helpful so long as these beats are recorded in leads MCL_1, MCL_6, V_1, or V_6, and preferably in both V_1 and V_6 or both MCL_1 and MCL_6.

5. Drew BJ, Scheinman MM. ECG criteria to distinguish between aberrantly conducted supraventricular tachycardia and ventricular

tachycardia: practical aspects for the immediate care setting. *Pacing Clin Electrophysiol.* **1995;18:1–15.**

Study Sample

Wide QRS tachycardias (n = 133) recorded from 112 patients undergoing a cardiac electrophysiologic study.

Comparison Studied

The standard 12-lead ECG recorded with electrodes on the torso to approximate lead placement with a bedside monitor was compared with the bedside monitoring leads MCL_1 and MCL_6.

Study Procedures

Tachycardia tracings were analyzed for the presence of findings that met currently available criteria for differentiating wide QRS tachycardias. These criteria were modified to make analysis more applicable to the bedside setting. Specific measurements of QRS intervals were rounded up to make measuring easier at the bedside. For example, a measurement of 30 milliseconds was rounded up to 40 milliseconds, or 0.04 seconds. Intracardiac leads were used to make the definitive diagnosis of supraventricular vs ventricular tachycardia.

Key Results

Ninety percent of wide QRS tachycardias were correctly diagnosed by using the 12-lead ECG and currently available criteria. Although the findings with the MCL_1 lead looked identical to those with the V1 lead during sinus rhythm, the MCL1 lead recorded clearly different QRS morphologies during wide QRS tachycardia 40% of the time and was statistically inferior to lead V1 for diagnosing ventricular tachycardia. Lead V1 was the best lead for showing atrioventricular dissociation and ventriculoatrial block (both of which favor ventricular tachycardia). The currently available criteria for differentiating wide QRS rhythms were reconfirmed with the following differences: (1) A QRS width of more than 0.16 second was more accurate than the currently accepted 0.14-second width for diagnosing ventricular tachycardia. Multiple leads are necessary for accurate measurement of QRS width. (2) A monophasic R wave in lead V1 was not diagnostic of ventricular tachycardia, although a taller left *rabbit ear* was.

Study Strengths and Weaknesses

This study showed that the established criteria for differentiating wide QRS rhythms can be used accurately at the bedside with conventional placement of ECG leads. Making this information applicable to bedside nurses in their clinical setting is a major strength of this study. The results reconfirm the usefulness of established criteria for differentiating wide QRS rhythms with the 12-lead ECG.

Clinical Implications

Because lead MCL_1 is inferior to lead V_1 for differentiating wide QRS rhythms, every effort should be made to use a 5-lead system and monitor in a true unipolar V_1 lead. A full 12-lead recording should be obtained whenever possible during wide QRS rhythms, because many of the criteria used require multiple leads for accurate analysis. Because ventricular tachycardia is more common than supraventricular tachycardia, when there is any doubt about the origin of a wide QRS tachycardia, the rhythm should be considered ventricular tachycardia until proved otherwise.

6. Drew BJ, Scheinman MM. Value of electrocardiographic leads MCL_1, MCL_6, and other selected leads in the diagnosis of wide QRS complex tachycardia. *J Am Coll Cardiol.* **1991;18:1025–1033.**

Study Sample

Wide QRS tachycardias (n = 121) were recorded from 92 patients during a cardiac electrophysiologic study.

Comparison Studied

Leads MCL_1 and MCL_6 were compared with leads V_1 and V_6 to assess the accuracy of using information obtained with these leads to diagnose wide QRS tachycardias. In addition, the new criterion used in the previous study (reference 5 in this bibliography), measurement of onset of QRS to tallest peak or nadir in lead V_6 or lead MCL_6, was assessed for its usefulness in accurately diagnosing wide QRS tachycardias.

Study Procedures

Information from leads MCL_1 and MCL_6, a conventional 12-lead ECG, and intracardiac leads were recorded in all patients during baseline rhythm and during wide complex tachycardia. The electrode wires for leads MCL_1 and V_1 were soldered together as were those for leads MCL_6 and V_6, because the same spot on the chest is required to record information from more than 1 lead. Findings obtained with leads MCL_1 and MCL_6 were compared with findings obtained with leads V_1 and V_6 by 2 observers who rated the QRS complexes as identical, similar, or clearly different. The MCL leads were also compared with the V leads by using well-established criteria for QRS morphology for differentiating wide QRS rhythms. Each of these QRS patterns was compared with the diagnosis based on findings obtained with intracardiac leads. To determine which leads were most valuable in diagnosing wide QRS tachycardias, a diagnosis of supraventricular tachycardia, ventricular tachycardia, or indeterminate tachycardia was made on the basis of findings on rhythm strips and compared with the diagnosis based on information obtained with intracardiac leads. The leads evaluated were those most commonly used for bedside monitoring: MCL_1, MCL_6, V_1, V_6, and II. These leads were evaluated singly and in various combinations for their accuracy in diagnosing wide QRS tachycardias.

Key Results

QRS complexes in leads MCL_1 and MCL_6 were comparable to those in leads V_1 and V_6 during baseline rhythm, but significant discrepancies occurred during ventricular tachycardia, especially between lead MCL_1 and lead V_1. These differences did not affect diagnostic accuracy. Measuring from onset of QRS to tallest peak or nadir in lead V_6 or lead MCL_6 was useful in distinguishing supraventricular tachycardia from ventricular tachycardia, and with this criterion, lead V_6 or lead MCL_6 was as useful as lead V_1 or lead MCL_1 for diagnosing wide QRS rhythms. Diagnostic accuracy with leads MCL_1, V_1, MCL_6, and V_6 was comparable and far superior to that with lead II. Combinations of MCL_1 + MCL_6, V_1 + V_6, V_1 + I + aVF, or V_1 + V_6 + I + aVF are superior to any single lead and to the routinely monitored combination of V_1 + II.

Study Strengths and Weaknesses

This study reconfirmed most of the previously published criteria for differentiating wide QRS complexes of both right and left bundle-branch block morphologies. The results validated using leads MCL_1 and MCL_6 as substitutes for leads V_1 and V_6 for bedside monitoring. They also validated using findings obtained with leads V_6 or MCL_6 to differentiate wide QRS tachycardias when early or late peaking in these leads is used as a criterion for diagnosis. A larger sample size might further clarify the discrepancy that occurred in this study between leads V_1 and MCL_1 during ventricular tachycardia.

Clinical Implications

For single-channel 3-lead monitors, lead MCL_1 or lead MCL_6 is most accurate for diagnosis of wide QRS tachycardias. For dual-channel 5-lead monitors, MCL_1 + MCL_6 is a good combination for diagnosing wide QRS tachycardias, but using it requires placing the electrodes in confusing positions on the thorax and eliminates the ability to scroll through the limb leads by using the lead-select button on the monitor.

7. Drew BJ, Ide B, Sparacino PS. Accuracy of bedside electrocardiographic monitoring: a report on current practices of critical care nurses. Heart Lung. 1991;20:597–607.

Study Sample

Randomly selected AACN members (n = 302).

Comparison Studied

A questionnaire was used to ask nurses to demonstrate placement of electrodes and attachment of lead wires for obtaining the single lead of choice for single-channel monitors or the two leads of choice for dual-channel monitors. All nurses were asked to demonstrate their technique for obtaining MCL_1 and MCL_6 leads, whether or not they routinely used these leads. Additional data about nursing practices regarding selection of leads and documentation of arrhythmia were also collected but were not reported.

Key Results

Seventy-four percent of critical care nurses in this study used lead II for single-channel monitoring. Eighty-seven percent used lead II plus lead V_1 (or MCL_1) for dual-channel monitoring. Sixty-three percent demonstrated incorrect technique for obtaining their lead of choice: incorrect placement of electrodes (59%), incorrect attachment of lead wires to electrodes (26%), and both incorrect placement of electrodes and incorrect attachment of lead wires (15%). Eighty-seven percent of nurses demonstrated incorrect technique for obtaining their 2 leads of choice for dual-channel monitoring: incorrect placement of electrodes (93%) and both incorrect placement of electrodes and incorrect attachment of lead wires (7%). Ninety-one percent demonstrated incorrect technique for obtaining lead MCL1, and 88% demonstrated incorrect technique for obtaining lead MCL6. Additional findings of this study showed that nursing routines and practices do not promote appropriate selection of leads, documentation of arrhythmia, or accurate placement of leads.

Study Strengths and Weaknesses

A major strength of the study is that it targeted bedside monitoring practices and showed areas of weakness in a majority of nurses' practice in this area. Weaknesses include a small sample size, inclusion of AACN members only, and inclusion of nurses other than those working in intensive care, cardiac care, or step-down units. Use of a questionnaire to assess practice is less accurate than direct observation of practice.

Clinical Implications

This study showed serious deficiencies in nursing education related to monitoring practices. Nursing education needs to include (1) the goals of monitoring for individual patients (ECG abnormalities and arrhythmias essential to detect based on the patient's clinical problem); (2) diagnostic criteria for recognizing arrhythmias and ECG abnormalities; (3) most valuable leads for bedside monitoring and proper placement of electrodes and attachment of lead wires to obtain these leads; and (4) strategies to promote better detection, documentation, and diagnosis of arrhythmias.

8. Thomason TR, Riegel B, Carlson B, Gocka I. Monitoring electrocardiographic changes:

results of a national survey. *J Cardiovasc Nurs.* **1995;9:1–9.**

Study Sample

Nurses (n = 882) who care for patients with acute myocardial infarction.

Study Procedures

A survey was used to ask nurses about their monitoring practices when caring for patients with acute myocardial infarction. Areas of interest included selection of leads, diagnosis of infarct evolution, and use of right precordial leads.

Key Results

The nurses indicated that when a single-channel monitor is used, lead II is still the lead most often selected (66.3%), and lead MCL_1 is the second choice (25.9%). When dual-channel monitors are used, the most commonly used combinations are leads II and MCL_1 (36.2%), and leads II and V_1 (26.2%). Only 20% of the respondents reported that they always modify lead selection on the basis of the location of the infarction, and 38.6% never do. Forty-six percent of the nurses responding correctly identified the definition of acute injury pattern on ECGs, 62.7% correctly identified the definition of ischemia, 73.9% correctly identified the definition of acute infarction, and 43.3% correctly identified all 3. Forty-three percent said that right precordial leads were not recorded in their unit; 7% said right precordial leads are used almost all the time in patients with inferior myocardial infarction.

Study Strengths and Weaknesses

This study looked at some important and interesting issues related to bedside monitoring, particularly the use of right precordial leads and the ability of nurses to recognize ischemia, injury, and infarction. A limitation is that nurses were not given an actual ECG to identify patterns of ischemia, injury, and infarction; they were only asked to match the word with the correct definition.

Clinical Implications

There continue to be deficiencies in the bedside monitoring practice of nurses working in monitored units. Nursing education related to monitoring practices needs to include (1) emphasis on proper placement of electrodes and selection of leads based on the patient's clinical situation, (2) use of V_1 monitoring strips in teaching basic arrhythmia classes so nurses become familiar with complexes recorded in that lead, and (3) discussion of the ECG criteria useful in rhythm identification and the superiority of lead V_1 over other leads in making accurate diagnoses, especially when the QRS is wide. Research findings related to monitoring (both detection of arrhythmia and ST-segment monitoring) can be dis-

seminated at the unit level by use of journal clubs, discussion on rounds, and posted articles for staff to read.

9. Drew BJ. Bedside electrocardiographic monitoring: state of the art for the 1990s. *Heart Lung.* 1991;20:610–623.

Description

This article reviews the ECG criteria for using ST-segment monitoring to differentiate wide QRS rhythms, diagnose bundle-branch block, and recognize ischemia after thrombolytic therapy or PTCA. Strategies to improve the quality of bedside ECG monitoring are suggested.

Clinical Implications

The authors offer the following suggestions: When choosing a monitoring lead, nurses should consider the goals of monitoring for each patient. They should determine what arrhythmias are likely to occur and consider if the patient is at risk for an ischemic event (eg, after PTCA or thrombolytic therapy). Good skin preparation techniques and accurate placement of leads and attachment of cables for chosen leads are essential. When receiving a patient from another unit, nurses should not assume that lead placement is accurate. Knowledge of the capabilities and limitations of the monitoring system being used and of proper techniques for working with the equipment is important. Alarm limits should be set so that arrhythmias will be documented on paper. Several examples of how to use alarm limits are given in the article.

Whenever possible, a 12-lead ECG should be used to document ST changes and sustained arrhythmias. A 12-lead ECG machine should be immediately available in every critical care unit, and unit policies should allow nurses to record ECGs without a physician's order or without relying on an ECG technician. Bedside monitors should be used to their maximum potential. If 2 or 3 leads are available for ECG monitoring, they should all be routinely used. If a true V_1 lead is available, it should be used instead of the substitute MCL_1 lead as the first choice and lead MCL_6 as the second choice. If 2 leads are available, lead V_1 should be used as the first one; the second lead should be chosen on the basis of the patient's clinical situation. Another useful dual-lead combination for patients likely to have wide QRS rhythms is leads MCL_1 and MCL_6 together. If 3 leads are available, a good combination is leads V_1, I, and aVF.

Nurses should know the ECG criteria for diagnosing arrhythmias of major concern. They should also know the ECG criteria for differentiating wide QRS rhythms, and quick reference information should be posted where it is easily available at the bedside for use when arrhythmias occur.

10. Drew BJ, Tisdale LA. ST-segment monitoring for coronary artery reocclusion following thrombolytic therapy and coronary

angioplasty: identification of optimal bedside monitoring leads. *Am J Crit Care.* **1993;2:280–292.**

Study Subjects

Adult cardiac patients (n = 27) who had acute myocardial infarction (2) or had PTCA (25).

Comparison Studied

The purpose of the study was to determine which of the limb leads provides the greatest sensitivity for detecting myocardial ischemia.

Study Procedures

Thirty episodes of acute ischemia in 27 patients were recorded by using a standard 12-lead ECG, and these patients were followed up with ST-segment monitoring in a cardiac care unit. In the patients who had PTCA, baseline ECGs were recorded before the procedure, and continuous 12-lead ECGs were recorded during balloon inflation and until ST segments normalized. ST segments were measured manually for all 12 leads at the time of greatest ST-segment deviation, and the findings were compared with baseline ST values. In the 2 patients who had myocardial infarction, the maximum ST deviation was measured on an ECG obtained before thrombolytic therapy and compared with the isoelectric PR segment. During follow-up, 18 patients were monitored in the cardiac care unit with a bedside monitor capable of measuring ST-segment deviation in 3 leads (1 precordial and 2 limb leads). Lead V_1 was used as the precordial lead; the limb leads were the 2 that showed greatest ST deviation during the ischemic episode.

Key Results

Ischemia of the right coronary artery was detected in all cases by using a single lead: lead III or lead aVF. Ischemia of the left anterior descending artery was best detected with precordial leads V_2, V_3, and V_4. The limb leads with greatest sensitivity for detection of ischemia were leads III and aVF. Ischemia in the circumflex artery was best detected with leads III, aVF, and V_2. In the group as a whole, the 2 best leads for detecting ischemia were leads III and aVF. The highest sensitivity of any lead combination for detecting ischemia of the left anterior descending artery was V_1 + aVF (79% sensitivity). The lead with the highest sensitivity for detecting ischemia in the circumflex artery was lead III or lead aVF (71% sensitivity). The lead with the highest sensitivity for detecting ischemia of the right coronary artery was lead III or lead aVF (100% sensitivity).

Study Strengths and Weaknesses

The sample size was small, and not all patients had bedside ST-segment monitoring. None of the 18 patients who had

ST-segment monitoring in the follow-up period had ischemia, so there was no direct evidence of the bedside monitor's ability to detect ischemia in these patients. Two patients did experience recurrent ischemia, but neither had bedside monitoring for ST-segment deviation. The study found no direct evidence that the bedside monitor would have picked up the ischemia in these patients, although a stat 12-lead ECG showed the same ischemic fingerprint as that obtained during PTCA. The study showed the best lead combinations and the best limb leads for detecting ischemia during the acute episode. This information is useful and has strong clinical implications for the use of bedside ST-segment monitoring.

Clinical Implications

When the ischemic fingerprint is not available, leads V_1 + III or V_1 + aVF are the best dual-lead combination for detecting arrhythmia and for ST-segment monitoring. When the choice is between lead III and lead aVF, the one with the tallest QRS complex should be used. If lead V_1 cannot be used, lead V_6 is the next best lead for monitoring arrhythmia. A good 3-lead combination is V_1 + I + aVF. A good 4-lead combination is V_1 + I + III + aVF.

11. **Mizutani M, Freedman SB, Barns E, et al. ST monitoring for myocardial ischemia during and after coronary angioplasty.** *Am J Cardiol.* **1990;66:389–393.**

Study Sample

Patients undergoing PTCA (n = 97).

Comparison Studied

Twelve-lead ECG monitoring was done during PTCA to determine the optimum lead or lead combination for detecting ST-segment deviation during acute ischemia. Patients were divided into 2 groups on the basis of evidence of ischemia during PTCA (chest pain, ST elevation, or both). Comparisons were made between the 2 groups in terms of clinical, angiographic, and hemodynamic subsets.

Study Procedures

Twelve-lead ECGs were recorded at 10-second intervals before and during each balloon inflation. Significant change in the ST segment was defined as 1 mm or more elevation or depression 60 milliseconds after the J point relative to the TP segment. In 50 patients who had ST elevation during PTCA, the lead that showed maximum ST elevation during PTCA was used to monitor the patients for a mean of 20 hours after PTCA.

Key Results

The most sensitive lead for detecting ST elevation was lead V_2 or lead V_3 for the left anterior descending artery, lead III for the circumflex artery, and lead III or lead aVF for the right coronary artery. The most sensitive lead for detecting ST depression was lead III for the left anterior descending artery, lead V_2 or lead V_3 for the circumflex artery, and lead V_2 for the right coronary artery. The sensitivity was 80% for the best single lead for each artery, 93% for the best 2 leads, and 100% for the best 3 leads.

Clinical Implications

The study indicates that use of a single lead is inadequate in monitoring for ischemia, but the use of 2 appropriate leads provides a sensitivity of 93%, and the use of 3 appropriate leads could replace the 12-lead ECG for monitoring during PTCA. These findings could also apply to postprocedure monitoring in the cardiac care unit.

12. Tisdale LA, Drew BJ. ST-segment monitoring for myocardial ischemia. *AACN Clin Issues.* 1993;4:34–43.

Description

This article reviews the pathophysiology of coronary artery reocclusion after PTCA or thrombolytic therapy, ST-segment changes indicative of ischemia, ST analysis software, and selection of leads for ST-segment monitoring.

Clinical Implications

Because the goals of ECG monitoring include recognition of arrhythmia and early recognition of ischemia, the best leads for each goal should be used. Lead V_1 is the best lead for monitoring arrhythmia and should be included in all lead combinations. The patient's ischemic fingerprint should be used to choose the leads for ST-segment monitoring. When no ischemic fingerprint is available, combinations of leads $V_1 + I + aVF$ offer several advantages.

13. Hebra JD. The nurse's role in continuous dysrhythmia monitoring. *AACN Clin Issues.* 1994;5:178–185.

Description

The author reviews current research on continuous bedside monitoring and lead selection and offers recommendations to improve monitoring practices.

Clinical Implications

Selection of leads should be based on the monitoring goals for each patient. Nurses should know proper placement of electrodes and proper attachment of lead wires to achieve the chosen lead. Proper skin preparation should include washing the site with soap and water and drying it vigorously to remove dead skin. Electrodes should be replaced every 48 hours to prevent drying of the electrode gel, and all patches should be replaced if one replacement is needed. At the start of each shift, nurses should confirm that lead wires are con-

nected properly, electrodes are in the proper locations, and the appropriate leads are selected for the patient. The monitoring lead on each rhythm strip should be indicated.

14. Drew BJ, Adams MG, Pelter MM, Wung SF. ST-segment monitoring with a derived 12-lead electrocardiogram is superior to routine CCU monitoring. *Am J Crit Care.* 1996;5:198–206.

Study Sample

Patients treated for angina or myocardial infarction in a cardiac care unit (n = 250).

Comparison Studied

The study compared the value of continuous, derived 12-lead ST-segment monitoring vs routine cardiac monitoring with leads V_1 and II.

Study Procedures

Patients were monitored continuously with leads V_1 and II with standard placement of leads in a 5-wire system and simultaneously with a continuous 12-lead ST-segment monitor that derives the 12-lead ECG from 6 electrodes placed on the thorax. The ST-segment monitor was programmed to alarm and store any ECG with an ST-segment deviation of 1 mm in 1 or more of the 12 leads. With every alarm, the nurse ran a dual channel rhythm strip of leads V_1 and II for comparison.

Key Results

Fifty-five patients had evidence of ischemia on the derived 12-lead ECG, and of these, 64% did not show evidence of ischemia in routine leads V_1 or II. Five patients with abrupt reocclusion of a coronary artery after PTCA had ischemic changes on the derived 12-lead ECG, and only 2 of them had ST changes on the routine monitoring leads. Seventy-five percent of patients with transient ischemia had no symptoms (silent ischemia). The incidence of serious complications was higher in patients with recurrent ischemia than in those without (17% vs 3%). Lengths of stay in the cardiac care unit and the hospital were twice as long for patients with recurrent ischemia as they were for patients without this complication.

Study Strengths and Weaknesses

The study showed the value of continuous 12-lead ECG monitoring in detecting ischemic episodes and illustrated the high incidence of silent ischemia, which can go undetected with conventional cardiac monitoring. It also addressed the high incidence of false alarms that can occur and stressed the need to evaluate the actual ECG and not just trends or graphic reports of ST-segment deviations. The routine leads V_1 and II were not programmed to monitor ST segments, so the study made no direct comparison of routine bedside ST-segment monitoring with the derived 12-lead

ECG ST-segment monitoring. The small number of patients with abrupt reocclusion after PTCA makes it difficult to evaluate using routine monitoring and the derived 12-lead ECG to detect this complication.

Clinical Implications

ST-segment monitoring is a useful tool for detecting recurrent ischemia, but it requires a clinician trained in interpreting the actual ECG and not just numerical or graphic trends, which often represent false-positive alarms. The high incidence of silent ischemia and the inadequacy of routine monitoring leads V_1 and lead II for detecting ischemia indicate the need for some type of ST-segment monitoring in units where patients at risk for ischemia are placed.

15. Drew BJ, Pelter MM, Adams MG, Wung SF, Chou TM, Wolfe CL. 12-lead ST-segment monitoring vs single-lead maximum ST-segment monitoring for detecting ongoing ischemia in patients with unstable coronary syndromes. *Am J Crit Care*. 1998;7:355–363.

Study Sample

Patients admitted to CCU with ischemic coronary events or following catheter-based coronary interventions (n = 422)

Study Procedures

Continuous 12-lead ST-segment monitoring was performed from the onset of myocardial infarction or during balloon inflation in catheter-based interventions until discharge. The derived 12-lead ECG was obtained using the EASI lead system. Computer-assisted techniques were used to determine which lead showed the maximum ST deviation during the acute ischemic event and what proportion of later ischemic events were associated with ST deviation in this lead.

Key Results

The lead with the maximum ST deviation could be determined in 312 patients (74%). During the monitoring period, 118 (28%) of the 312 patients had a total of 463 ischemic events, 80% of which were silent. Of 377 ischemic events in which a maximum ST lead was detected, 159 (42%) did not show ST deviation in that maximum ST lead during ischemia (sensitivity 58%). The most commonly used monitoring leads II and V_1 showed ST changes in only 33% of ischemic events.

Study Strengths and Weaknesses

The study demonstrated the value of using all 12 leads for continuous monitoring of patients with acute coronary syndromes. In this study, even identification of the lead with the maximum ST deviation and monitoring in that lead without the benefit of 12-lead monitoring would have missed 42% of ischemic events. It also demonstrated the high incidence

of silent ischemia that occurs in these patients and reconfirmed other studies that have shown that lead II and V_1, commonly used for arrhythmia monitoring, are even less sensitive than the maximum ST lead for detecting ischemia. These results cannot be used to determine whether patients would have better outcomes if recurrent ischemic events were more accurately detected.

Clinical Implications

These results imply that monitoring in all 12 ECG leads for changes in the ST segment is necessary to accurately detect ongoing ischemia in patients with unstable coronary syndromes. If continuous 12 lead monitoring is not available, using the lead with maximum ST deviation for ST-segment monitoring is better than relying on leads II or V_1 but can still miss as many as 42% of ischemic events.

16. Drew BJ, Krucoff MW. Multilead ST-segment monitoring in patients with acute coronary syndromes: a consensus statement for healthcare professionals. *Am J Crit Care*. 1999;8:372–386.

Description

This consensus document provides clinically practical guidelines for optimal ST-segment monitoring in patients with acute coronary syndromes. A working group of key nurses and physicians who had published articles on ST-segment monitoring met and reached consensus on who should and should not have ST-segment monitoring, goals, and time frames for ST-segment monitoring in various diagnostic categories; what ECG leads should be monitored; what equipment requirements are needed; what strategies improve accuracy and clinical usefulness of ST-segment monitoring; and what knowledge and skills are required for safe and effective ST-segment monitoring.

Clinical Implications

The document provides answers to several questions that can guide hospitals in providing optimum patient care. Two of the more important questions are:

1. Who should have ST-segment monitoring? Patients with unstable angina and ST elevation or non-ST elevation MI are highest priority. Others who may benefit include patients with chest pain prompting a visit to the emergency department, catheter-based interventions, coronary vasospasm, cardiac surgery, high risk patients with noncardiac surgery.
2. What ECG leads should be monitored? Continuous 12-lead ECG monitoring is recommended. The best lead for detecting occlusion of the right coronary artery is lead III. The best leads for detecting left anterior descending coronary artery occlusion are V_2 and V_3. If continuous 12-lead monitoring is not available, monitoring the lead

that showed peak ST-segment elevation during the acute ischemic event is useful for detecting reocclusion of the infarct-related artery or the treated artery following PCI. The most valuable 2-lead combination if 12-lead monitoring is not available is lead III and V_3. The best 3-lead combination is lead III, V_3, and V_5 if multiple V leads are available.

17. Drew BJ, Califf RM, Funk M, et al. Practice standards for electrocardiographic monitoring in hospital settings. *Circulation*. 2004;110:2721–2746.

Description

This expert consensus paper is a comprehensive document outlining recommendations for bedside arrhythmia monitoring, ST-segment monitoring and QT-interval monitoring in pediatric and adult patients in the hospital. In the absence of published clinical trials in the area of hospital cardiac monitoring, this document provides expert opinions based upon clinical experience and related research in the field of electrocardiography. Recommendations follow the rating system used by the American College of Cardiology Emergency Cardiac Care Committee and consist of the following categories:

Class I: Cardiac monitoring is indicated in most, if not all, patients in this group.

Class II: Cardiac monitoring may be of benefit in some patients but is not considered essential for all.

Class III: Cardiac monitoring is not indicated because the patient's risk of a serious event is so low that monitoring is not of therapeutic benefit.

Clinical Implications

This document provides guidelines for patient selection for cardiac arrhythmia monitoring, ST-segment monitoring, and QT-interval monitoring that serve as a guide for hospitals in writing policies related to which patients should be monitored as well as on what type of unit this monitoring should occur (emergency department, critical care versus telemetry). It also provides a discussion about cardiac monitoring lead systems and compares standard monitoring lead systems with derived 12-lead ECG systems and can serve as a guide for equipment selection by hospitals. Staff training, qualifications of staff, and documentation related to cardiac monitoring are discussed and can serve as guides to educa-

tors and hospitals in providing orientation and verifying competency in cardiac monitoring.

OTHER REFERENCES

1. Dracup K. *Meltzer's Intensive Coronary Care,* 5th ed. Norwalk, Conn: Appleton & Lange; 1995.
2. Dasher LA, Slye DA. *ECG, Arrhythmia and ST Segment Analysis.* Redmond, Wash: Spacelabs Medical, Inc; 1994.
3. Drew BJ. Bedside electrocardiogram monitoring. *AACN Clin Issues.*1993;4:25–33.
4. Wellens HJ, Bar FW, Lie KI. The value of the electrocardiogram in the differential diagnosis of a tachycardia with a widened QRS complex. *Am J Med.* 1978;64:27–33.
5. Sandler JA, Marriott HJL. The differential morphology of anomalous ventricular complexes of RBBB-type in lead V_1: ventricular ectopy versus aberration. *Circulation.* 1965;31:551–556.
6. Krucoff MW, Jackson YR, Kehoe MK, Kent KM. Quantitative and qualitative ST-segment monitoring during and after PTCA. *Circulation.* 1990;81(3 suppl):IV 20–26.
7. Stablein A, von Polnitz A, Reuschel-Janetchek E, von Arnim T, Hofling B. Multiple lead monitoring during and after PTCA. *Eur Heart J.* 1989;10(suppl G):9–12.
8. Fesmire FM, Smith EE. Continuous 12-lead ECG monitoring in the emergency department. *Am J Emerg Med.* 1993;11:54–60.
9. Veldkamp RF, Green CL, Wilkins ML, et al. Comparison of continuous ST-segment recovery analysis with methods using static ECG for noninvasive assessment during acute myocardial infarction. Thrombolysis and Angioplasty in Myocardial Infarction (TAMI) 7 Study Group. *Am J Cardiol.* 1994;73:1069–1074.
10. Medical Device Safety Report: Risk of electrical shock from patient monitoring cables and electrode lead wires. *Health Devices.* 1993;22:301.
11. Drew BJ. Using cardiac leads the right way. *Nursing.* May 1992:50–54
12. Adams-Hamoda MG, Caldwell MA, Stotts NA, Drew BJ. Factors to consider when analyzing 12-lead electrocardiograms for evidence of acute myocardial ischemia. *Am J Crit Care.* 2003;12:9–16.

Respiratory Waveforms Monitoring

Suzanne M. Burns, RN, MSN, RRT, ACNP, CCRN, FAAN, FCCM, FAANP

CHAPTER TWO

Respiratory Waveforms Monitoring

CASE STUDY

Ms West, a 63-year-old woman, was admitted to the medical intensive care unit (MICU) after 1 week of intermittent fever, nausea with emesis, and a productive cough associated with increased dyspnea. She has a history of chronic obstructive pulmonary disease associated with tobacco use. Soon after admission, her body temperature increased to 39°C (102°F) and she became increasingly short of breath. Her respiratory rate was 32 breaths/min and labored, and analysis of arterial blood gases shows respiratory acidosis, with pH = 7.28, $PaCO_2$ = 76 mm Hg, and PaO_2 = 56 mm Hg. The bronchodilator albuterol was administered, but there was no change in respiratory status. Ms West was given midazolam and succinylcholine and electively intubated for mechanical ventilation. The initial ventilator settings were as follows: Fraction of inspired oxygen (FIO_2) = 0.60, mode of ventilation = assist control at a rate of 15, tidal volume (V_T) = 600 mL, and positive end-expiratory pressure (PEEP) = 5 cm of H_2O. Because Ms West was paralyzed to facilitate intubation, the initial airway pressure waveforms do not show any spontaneous effort (negative deflections) (Figure 2.1).

Later that afternoon, Ms West was alert and able to mouth words, indicating relief of her dyspnea. Spontaneous respirations occurred intermittently with positioning and suctioning. The ventilator settings appeared to be appropriate as indicated by clinical assessment and by pressure waveform analysis, which demonstrated patient initiated breaths at a reasonable respiratory rate (Figure 2.2).

CASE DISCUSSION

Monitoring respiratory waveforms is a convenient method of visually assessing a patient's ventilatory tolerance. In Ms

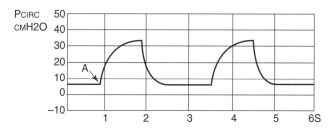

Figure 2.1 Ventilator-initiated mandatory (volume) breaths. Note that no spontaneous effort, which would be a negative deflection prior to the ventilator breath (A), is present prior to mandatory breath.

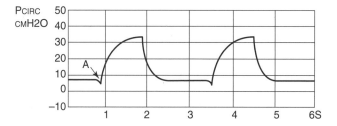

Figure 2.2 Patient-initiated volume breaths. A pressure deflection (A) indicating spontaneous effort is present prior to delivery of the volume breaths.

West's case, arterial blood gases were analyzed to confirm the clinical impression. The results were pH = 7.46, $PaCO_2$ = 33 mm Hg, and PaO_2 = 110 mm Hg. On the basis of these values, the decision was made to decrease the assist-control rate to 10. Throughout the ensuing shift, a brief analysis of the respiratory waveforms available on the ventilator verified that Ms West was synchronous with the ventilator.

The next day, Ms West returned to the MICU following a nuclear medicine study. She was short of breath, wheezing, and her respiratory rate was in the 30s. Routine nursing measures (such as suctioning to alleviate dyspnea) were performed, and pneumothorax was ruled out. However, no appreciable change in status occurred. It is thought that Ms West was anxious and that her anxiety had resulted in an increased respiratory rate, high minute ventilation and auto-PEEP. The respiratory flow waveforms were evaluated. It is noted that the expiratory limb of the flow waveform did not return to baseline before the next volume breath was delivered, confirming the presence of auto-PEEP (Figure 2.3). Intravenous midazolam was administered and Ms West was given an albuterol treatment. Within 3 minutes, her status improved, and her respiratory rate decreased to 10 breaths/min. As she began to awaken from the sedation, she was switched to pressure support (PS) ventilation at a pressure level of 15 cm H_2O (Figure 2.4). Her spontaneous rate was 18 and tidal volumes were approximately 500 mL. She was comfortable. The following day, Ms West was successfully extubated following a 1-hour trial of continuous positive airway pressure.

While many more respiratory waveforms were available on Ms West's ventilator, the clinicians focused on the use of pressure-time and flow-time waveforms. By using these

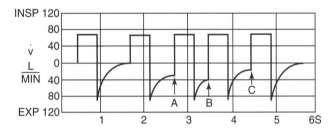

Figure 2.3 Determining the presence of auto-PEEP using flow-time waveforms. Auto-PEEP is the presence of positive pressure in the lungs at the end of exhalation. It is a result of inadequate expiratory time relative to the patient's condition. In this case, the expiratory portion of the flow waveforms (the portion below the baseline) does not return to baseline (waveforms 2, 3, and 4), indicating the presence of auto-PEEP.

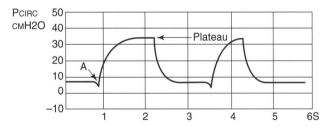

Figure 2.4 Pressure support ventilation. Patient-initiated breaths that rise to a plateau and display varying inspiratory times indicate pressure supported breaths.

waveform displays, they were quickly able to assess patient-ventilator synchrony and the presence of auto-PEEP. By using the waveforms, interventions such as ventilator adjustments and the use of bronchodilators were quickly provided.

GENERAL DESCRIPTION

Respiratory waveforms consist of breath-to-breath configurations of pressure, flow, and volume parameters. These 3 parameters are graphically displayed over time (pressure-time, flow-time, volume-time) or in "loop" configurations (pressure-volume and flow-volume). Most ventilator systems available today provide the graphics by means of a screen on the top of the ventilator and provide the clinician with a menu of options related to the display of the waveforms.

Much information may be gleaned by analyzing respiratory waveforms. Though the actual configurations of the waveforms vary slightly between ventilators, an understanding of the concepts related to these graphic respiratory representations is helpful and can be applied regardless of the ventilator system. To that end, the protocol describes various pressure, volume, and flow waveforms and potential applications.

Respiratory waveforms may be used to visually observe various interactions between a patient's spontaneous effort and ventilator mode settings. Thus, patient-ventilator dyssynchrony is quickly detected. Additional uses include the identification of ventilator modes, graphic detection of the presence of auto-PEEP, evaluation of compliance and resistance, improved accuracy in the measurement of hemodynamic values, and assessment of *breakthrough* respiratory efforts when chemical muscle relaxants are being used. These applications are described in the protocol.

As noted previously, respiratory waveform graphics are commonly integrated into new ventilator systems and are provided via a screen mounted on top of the ventilator. In addition, interaction between the ventilators and bedside physiologic monitoring systems is possible by means of a cable connection. The reader is referred to the specific ventilator user reference manual for detailed information on this application.

However, even ventilators that do not come with respiratory waveform graphics options may be adapted to display a pressure-time waveform continuously. This is called continuous airway pressure monitoring (CAPM). No expensive or special equipment is required for CAPM since the components of the system are common to virtually all critical care environments. This application and others are described in detail in the protocol.

ACCURACY

Respiratory waveforms may be continuously displayed and may be graphed. Damping of the waveforms occurs with leaks in the system, accumulation of condensation (moisture), and accumulation of airway secretions.

COMPETENCY

Competency requirements related to the use of respiratory waveform graphic displays consist of the ability to:

1. accurately set up the system so that the desired waveform configurations appear, and
2. correctly interpret the waveforms when displayed.

Setup

A demonstration–return demonstration competency is appropriate. The outcome of the demonstration is the appearance of the desired waveforms. The reader is referred to the product manufacturer's guidelines for specific setup procedures. In the case of CAPM, the pressure-time waveform should appear on the bedside monitoring system.

Interpretation of Waveforms

Personnel can become familiar with the waveforms produced by the various modes of ventilation by reviewing the concepts inherent in positive-pressure (ventilator) and negative-pressure (spontaneous) breathing. Knowing the difference between volume and pressure ventilation is important so that the differences in waveforms can be understood and accurately interpreted.

Competency verification depends on how the waveforms are used clinically and on the policies of individual institutions and critical care units. For example, if a pressure-time waveform is required to be graphed simultaneously with a pulmonary artery (PA) tracing in order to document end-expiration, the competency may be verified in conjunction with verification of competencies in measuring PA pressures.

FUTURE RESEARCH

Although monitoring of respiratory waveforms is increasingly present on ventilators, its usefulness has yet to be established. Many simply ignore the waveforms as just another "bell and whistle." Studies are needed to determine the efficacy of using the waveforms as a means of assessing such things as patient ventilator synchrony and auto-PEEP. To date, the waveforms are useful adjuncts to other assessment techniques, and usefulness is dependent on accurate interpretation. Because the waveforms may be graphed, they are especially useful to researchers for documentation purposes.

CLINICAL RECOMMENDATIONS

The rating scales for the Level of Recommendation column range from I to VI, with levels indicated as follows: I, manufacturer's recommendation only; II, theory based, no research data to support recommendations, recommendations from expert consensus group may exist; III, laboratory data only, no clinical data to support recommendations; IV, limited clinical studies to support recommendations; V, clinical studies in more than 1 or 2 different populations and situations to support recommendations; VI, clinical studies in a variety of patient populations and situations to support recommendations.

Period of Use	Recommendation	Rationale for Recommendation	Level of Recommendation	Supporting References	Comments
Selection of patients	Respiratory waveform monitoring may be especially helpful to monitor mechanically ventilated adult or pediatric patients on volume or pressure modes of mechanical ventilation. Waveform monitoring is generally less useful for evaluating high-frequency or oscillating modes. Because respiratory waveform monitoring is noninvasive, undetectable by the patient, and does not interfere with normal ventilator function, no special patient considerations are required for its use. Once the visual display is set up, a continuous visual display of selected waveforms is available and may be graphed (depending on the equipment).		III: Laboratory data only, no clinical data to support recommendations (this is the level appropriate to all recommendations listed unless otherwise stated)	See Annotated Bibliography: 1–8	Because respiratory waveform graphics are so prevalent in critical care it is important that critical care clinicians understand the theory and concepts related to the potential application of the technology. To date, there has been no research linking such monitoring to clinical outcomes.
	Commonly available waveform graphics on "newer ventilators" include: pressure-time, flow-time, volume-time, and "loop" configurations (pressure-volume and flow-volume loops).	Respiratory waveform monitoring is well grounded in the pathophysiologic principles of airway and pleural pressures. However, most of the potential applications of waveform monitoring are theoretical and fit in the category of applied science. Though they are useful in clinical practice, there are no studies demonstrating the relationship between clinical outcomes and the use of waveform monitoring.			
	While respiratory waveform monitoring has many potential applications, some of the most common and useful in the critical care unit include:				
	1. Identification of modes of ventilation.	Regardless, respiratory waveform monitoring is noninvasive, relatively easy to use and interpret, and is available on most new ventilators. The ventilator graphic displays vary between ventilators but the concepts are similar.			
	2. Evaluation of patient/ventilator synchrony.				
	3. Detection of auto-Positive End-Expiratory Pressure (PEEP) and air leaks.				

Period of Use	Recommendation	Rationale for Recommendation	Level of Recommendation	Supporting References	Comments
Selection of patients (continued)	4. Evaluation of changes in compliance and resistance. 5. Identification of end-expiration during hemodynamic monitoring. 6. Monitoring of spontaneous respiratory effort when muscle relaxants are being used. Recommended selected uses of the waveforms are found with each application below. **1. Identifying Ventilator Modes** **Ventilator modes** Identifying the mode of ventilation is commonly done using *pressure-time*, *flow-time*, and *volume-time* waveforms. (Figures 2.5, 2.6, 2.7)	*Pressure-time* waveform monitoring can be done using any ventilator (separate from the graphic packages available on current ventilators). With this system the pressure-time waveform is displayed on the bedside monitoring system using standard hemodynamic/arterial line monitoring equipment, which is adapted to the bedside monitoring system and the patient's ventilator circuit (described in the application section). A continuous, real-time pressure-time waveform is the result and is called Continuous Airway Pressure Monitoring or CAPM.			

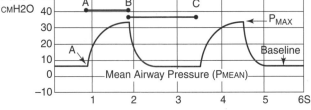

Figure 2.5 Typical pressure-time waveform. Inspiration is indicated as a rise in pressure (A to B in the figure), called an *accelerating* pressure waveform. Peak inspiratory pressure (Peak) appears as the highest point of the curve. Exhalation begins at the end of inspiration and continues until the next inspiration (B to C in the figure). The baseline is above zero, indicating the presence of PEEP.

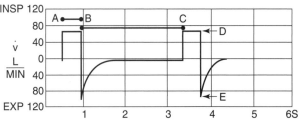

Figure 2.6 Flow-time waveforms. Flow refers to volume over time and is generally expressed in liters per minute (L/min). Inspiration is represented above the baseline and expiration below. A to B represents inspiratory time and expiratory time is seen from B to C. The highest expiratory flow rate (peak expiratory flow) is represented by E. This flow waveform is from a volume breath and is referred to as a *square* flow waveform.

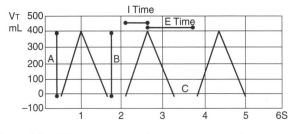

Figure 2.7 Volume-time waveforms. A represents inspiratory volume while B represents expiratory volume. Inspiratory and expiratory times are noted.

Period of Use	Recommendation	Rationale for Recommendation	Level of Recommendation	Supporting References	Comments
Selection of patients (continued)	Understanding essential concepts related to volume and pressure modes is required for accurate interpretation.				
	With volume modes of ventilation, volume is stable but airway pressure is dependent on changes in lung compliance and/or airways resistance. With pressure modes, pressure is stable and the volume varies.				
	Volume modes				
	Volume modes are associated with *accelerating pressure* waveforms (Figure 2.5), because pressure gradually builds as the volume of gas is delivered. Flow waveforms are generally a *square* configuration (Figure 2.6) because flow is stable throughout the breath. Examples include the following:				
	Assist-control (A/C) or assist mandatory ventilation (AMV): In this mode, a control or set rate and volume of gas are selected. Each time a spontaneous effort occurs, the ventilator delivers a breath at the control volume. In the assist-control mode, when the patient is breathing spontaneously, a negative deflection occurs before the *assisted* breath is delivered. The spacing between the waveforms may be irregular (Figure 2.8).				
	Intermittent mandatory ventilation (IMV) or synchronized mandatory ventilation (SIMV): In this mode, a mandatory number of ventilator breaths at a predetermined volume are selected. Between the mandatory breaths, spontaneous breathing occurs at a patient-determined rate and volume (Figure 2.9).				

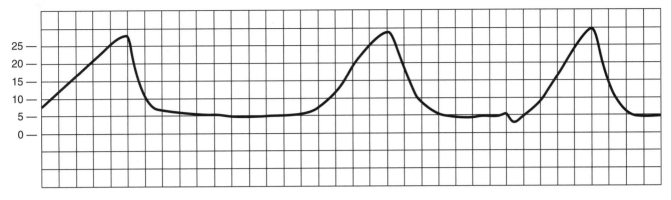

Figure 2.8 Assist-control ventilation with occasional spontaneous breaths. Note negative deflection indicating spontaneous patient effort.

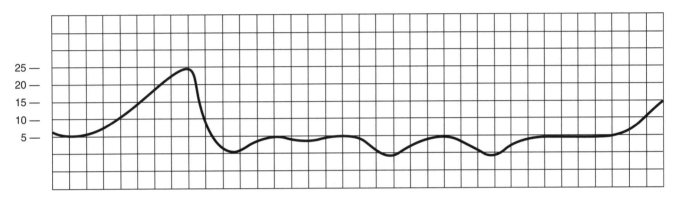

Figure 2.9 Intermittent mandatory ventilation with spontaneous respiratory effort by the patient. Note negative deflections.

Period of Use	Recommendation	Rationale for Recommendation	Level of Recommendation	Supporting References	Comments
Selection of patients (continued)	In the SIMV mode, the mandatory volume breaths may occur at irregularly spaced intervals, because the ventilator waits to give the mandatory breath in synchrony with the patient.				
	Pressure modes				
	With pressure modes, a high flow of gas is delivered until a predetermined pressure is reached. The pressure is maintained throughout inspiration and the associated waveform is called a *square pressure waveform* (Figure 2.10). Flow is initially high but tapers as the chest fills. The associated flow waveform is called a *decelerating* flow waveform (Figure 2.11).				

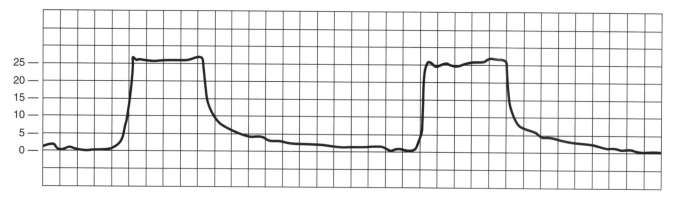

Figure 2.10   Pressure-support ventilation. Note square waveforms.

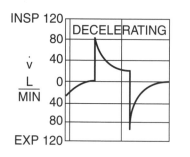

Figure 2.11   *Decelerating* flow waveform associated with pressure breaths.

Period of Use	Recommendation	Rationale for Recommendation	Level of Recommendation	Supporting References	Comments
Selection of patients (continued)	Examples include the following: *Pressure-support ventilation (PSV):* In this mode, patient-initiated breaths are augmented with a high flow of gas at a predetermined pressure. The patient controls the rate, volume, and inspiratory time (Figure 2.10). *Pressure-controlled/ inverse-ratio ventilation (PCIRV):* This mode is actually 2 modes in combination: pressure-controlled breaths at a set rate in conjunction with an inverse inspiratory-to-expiratory ratio (inspiration equal to or longer than expiration) (Figure 2.12).				

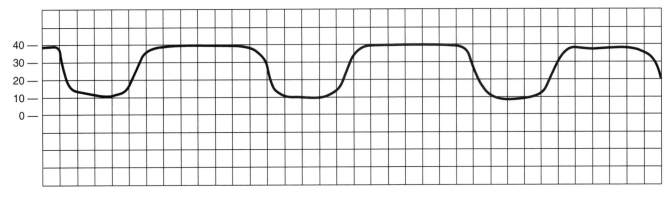

Figure 2.12 Pressure-controlled/inverse-ratio ventilation, 2:1 ratio. Note prolonged inspiratory time.

Period of Use	Recommendation	Rationale for Recommendation	Level of Recommendation	Supporting References	Comments
Selection of patients (continued)	*Volume-guaranteed pressure modes:* Some ventilators provide an option that allows a pre-selected volume to be *guaranteed* while providing the breath as a pressure breath. Waveforms vary, but the principles associated with detection of pressure (square) vs volume (accelerated) modes apply (Figures 2.13 and 2.14). Refer to the product manufacturer's operating manual to determine whether your equipment provides these modes.				

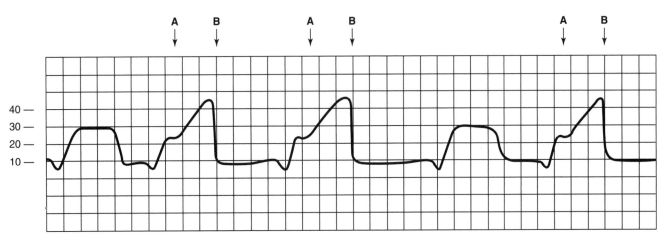

Figure 2.13 Volume-guaranteed pressure ventilation. Note how breaths 2, 3, and 5 start as pressure breaths (square, A) and end as volume breaths (accelerating, B). The volume is guaranteed.

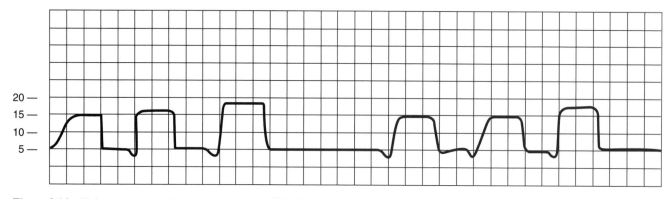

Figure 2.14   Volume-guaranteed pressure ventilation. With this particular ventilatory system, which differs from that used for Figure 13, the pressure level is automatically increased in a stepwise fashion to maintain volume.

Period of Use	Recommendation	Rationale for Recommendation	Level of Recommendation	Supporting References	Comments
Selection of patients (continued)	**Mixed modes** Volume and pressure modes of ventilation are commonly mixed (ie, IMV and PSV). When these 2 modes are used in combination, pressure and flow waveforms represent both volume and pressure breaths (Figures 2.15–2.17). **2. Patient-ventilator synchrony** When ventilators cannot deliver breaths as fast as the patient requires, asynchrony develops and is evident in the waveform. These changes in waveform configuration may indicate the need to change the mode of ventilation, adjust the inspiratory flow, shorten the inspiratory time, or sedate the				

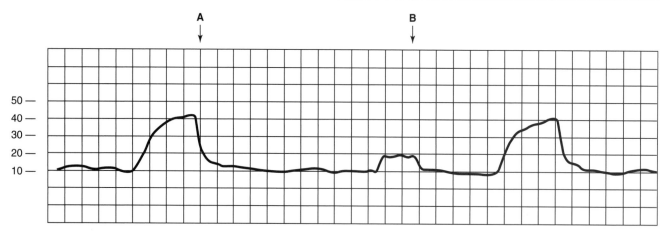

Figure 2.15   Mixed modes: intermittent mandatory (volume breath = A) and pressure-support (pressure breath = B) ventilation.

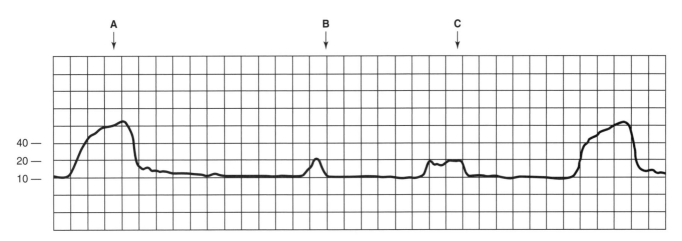

Figure 2.16 Mixed modes: intermittent mandatory (volume breath = A) and pressure-support (pressure breath = C) ventilation. Waveform B is an example of poor inspiratory effort on pressure-support ventilation. The volume associated with this breath is quite small.

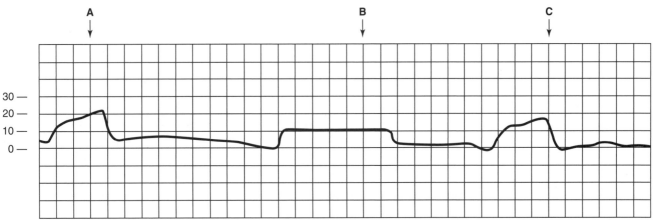

Figure 2.17 Mixed modes: intermittent mandatory (waveforms A and C) and pressure-support (waveform B) ventilation. Note the long inspiratory time associated with the pressure-support breath. This patient has a cuff leak. (Expiratory cycle of pressure-support ventilation begins only when the ventilator senses a decreased flow.)

Period of Use	Recommendation	Rationale for Recommendation	Level of Recommendation	Supporting References	Comments
Selection of patients (continued)	patient (Figures 2.18 and 2.19). While dys-synchrony can be seen in all waveforms, pressure-time waveforms are generally all that is necessary. **3. Auto-PEEP and leaks** Auto-PEEP occurs when not all the tidal volume is exhaled before the next breath. Auto-PEEP is common with long inspiratory times, short expiratory times, high minute ventilation requirements, small diameter endotracheal tubes, in patients with COPD and asthma,				

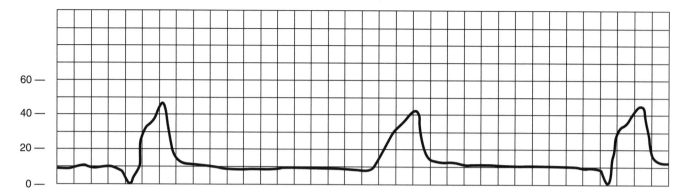

Figure 2.18   Patient-ventilator asynchrony in a patient receiving assist-control ventilation. The first and third waveforms indicate that the patient's requirement for inspiratory flow exceeds the flow provided by the ventilator. Thus, the waveforms lose the smooth accelerating shape associated with volume breaths.

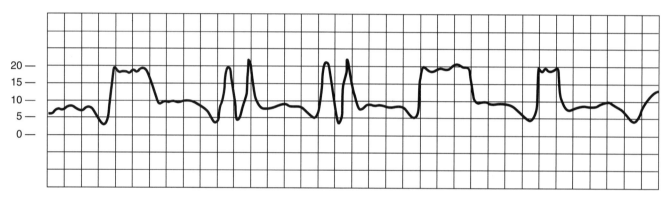

Figure 2.19   Patient-ventilator asynchrony. The patient was hiccuping while receiving pressure-support ventilation. The short, choppy waveforms indicate that the patient is not inspiring fully. Thus, the breaths are inadequate.

Period of Use	Recommendation	Rationale for Recommendation	Level of Recommendation	Supporting References	Comments
Selection of patients (continued)	when excess water condenses in the circuit, and in the elderly.				
	Auto-PEEP can be observed on a *pressure-time* waveform during an end-expiratory hold maneuver. The maneuver consists of activating the end-expiratory hold button at the end of expiration (just before inspiration).				Detection of auto-PEEP is difficult if the patient is agitated or breathing rapidly. Sedatives and paralytic agents may be necessary.
	If auto-PEEP is present, the baseline pressure increases during the maneuver (Figure 2.20).				
	If CAPM is being used, the bedside monitoring system displays in millimeters of mercury. Thus the units must be converted from millimeters of mercury to centimeters of water to				

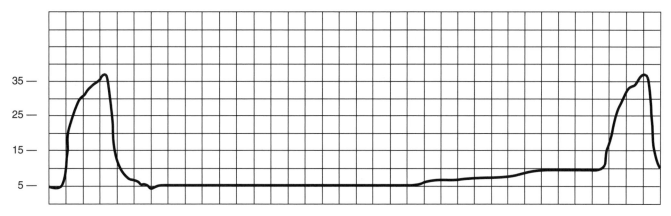

Figure 2.20 Auto-PEEP. Note the elevated end-expiratory pressure of 5 cm H_2O (arrow) above the set PEEP. Total PEEP is equal to 10 mmHg (5 set PEEP and 5 auto PEEP).

Period of Use	Recommendation	Rationale for Recommendation	Level of Recommendation	Supporting References	Comments
Selection of patients (continued)	*determine the exact amount (1.36 × value in millimeters of mercury = value in centimeters of water). This is not necessary with the graphic displays connected to the ventilator because they use cm H_2O as the units of measure.*				
	The expiratory limb of the *flow-time* waveform can also be evaluated to determine the presence of auto-PEEP. In this case the expiratory limb of the waveform will not return to baseline before the next breath is delivered (Figure 2.21). The flow-time waveform is also very helpful to assess the effectiveness of interventions to offset auto-PEEP such as the use of bronchodilators (Figure 2.22).				Remember to disconnect any in-line continuous flow aerosol devices before attempting the measurement because the flow used to power the aerosol will artificially elevate the pressure waveform baseline.

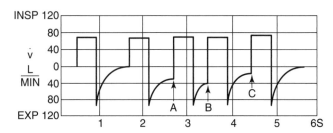

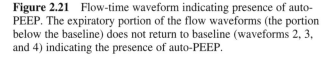

Figure 2.21 Flow-time waveform indicating presence of auto-PEEP. The expiratory portion of the flow waveforms (the portion below the baseline) does not return to baseline (waveforms 2, 3, and 4) indicating the presence of auto-PEEP.

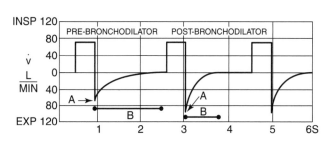

Figure 2.22 Evaluating bronchodilator response. Comparison of pre- and post-bronchodilator peak expiratory flow rates (A) and the time required for the expiratory limb of the flow waveform to return to baseline (B) demonstrate a positive response to bronchodilator therapy.

Period of Use	Recommendation	Rationale for Recommendation	Level of Recommendation	Supporting References	Comments
Selection of patients (continued)	With both air leaks and air trapping, volume delivery may not be accurate. The volume-time waveform demonstrates the disparity between volume delivered and volume exhaled (Figure 2.23). **Detection of changes in compliance or resistance** The *respiratory loops* are especially helpful to monitor changes in compliance and resistance. While orientation to the loops is a bit more confusing than the simpler pressure-time, flow-time, and volume-time waveforms, a brief orientation to the measurement units on the graphics helps to orient the clinician. *Pressure-volume loops* Pressure-volume loops vary dependent on whether the breath is a spontaneous (negative pressure) breath or a mandatory (positive pressure) ventilator breath. Spontaneous effort is reflected on the negative portion of the horizontal axis and mandatory ventilator breaths on the right (Figures 2.24–2.26).				

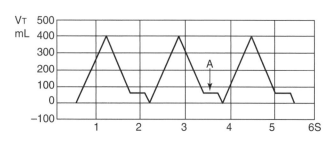

Figure 2.23 Air trapping or leaks noted in a volume-time waveform. Exhalation, A, does not return to zero. A disparity between volume in and volume out exists with both air trapping and leaks.

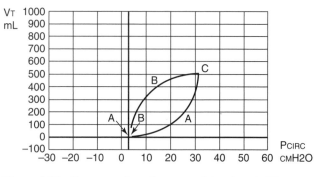

Figure 2.24 Pressure volume loop: mandatory breath. The loops are plotted in a counterclockwise direction, starting at the baseline (or PEEP level) with inspiration being drawn first (A), then expiration (B), C reflects peak inspiratory pressure.

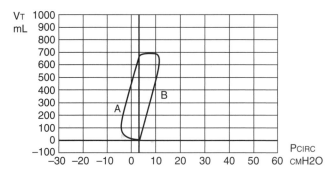

Figure 2.25 Pressure-volume loop: spontaneous breath. With spontaneous breaths the loop is plotted in a clockwise direction with A representing inspiration and B representing expiration.

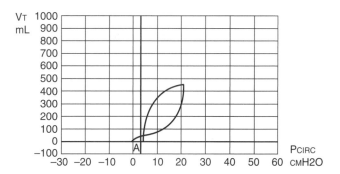

Figure 2.26 Pressure-volume loop: patient-initiated ventilator breath. In this waveform note the slight deflection (A) on the left side of the graph indicating patient spontaneous effort that triggers the ventilator breath (an example is the assist-control mode of ventilation).

Period of Use	Recommendation	Rationale for Recommendation	Level of Recommendation	Supporting References	Comments
Selection of patients (continued)	Assessment of changes in compliance and resistance are possible with pressure-volume loops, especially if the loops have been observed over time. *Compliance* Because greater pressure is required to distend a non-compliant lung, the slope of the pressure-volume loop will shift to the right and down (ie, a greater pressure is required to obtain a given volume) (Figures 2.27 and 2.28).				

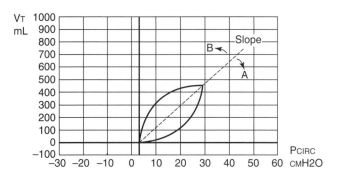

Figure 2.27 Pressure-volume loop: assessing compliance. The slope (or steepness) of the loop reflects the relationship of volume and pressure. A change in the slope of the loop indicates changes in compliance (A and B). A move towards A is a decrease in compliance, while a move of the slope towards B indicates improved compliance.

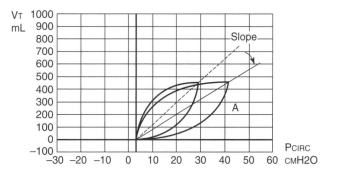

Figure 2.28 Pressure-volume loop: decreased compliance. The slope in this loop has moved down towards A. More pressure is required to deliver the same volume; compliance is decreased.

Period of Use	Recommendation	Rationale for Recommendation	Level of Recommendation	Supporting References	Comments
Selection of patients (continued)	*Resistance* With increased airway resistance, it is difficult to move volume down the airway. Thus the beginning portion of the loop will reflect an increase in pressure and is referred to as increased bowing (Figure 2.29). ***Flow-volume loops*** Flow-volume loops graph expiration first followed by exhalation. These loops are helpful in assessing the effect of bronchodilator therapy on peak flow (Figures 2.30 and 2.31). **Interpretation of hemodynamic measurements** Simultaneous monitoring of a *pressure-time* waveform and PA pressures provides a clear visual representation of end-expiration so that accurate standardized measurements of PA pressure can be made.			Annotated Bibliography: 1, 4, 5, 6	

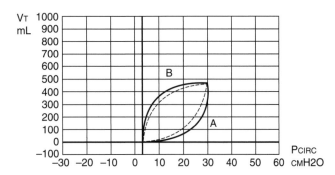

Figure 2.29 Pressure-volume loop: assessing resistance. Resistance to flow (ie, airways resistance) is demonstrated by increased "bowing" on the inspiratory curve of the waveform (A) and suggests inspiratory resistance to flow. Bowing of the expiratory curve (B) is indicative of expiratory resistance.

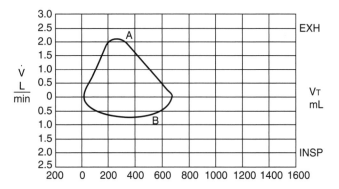

Figure 2.30 Flow-volume loop. In flow-volume loops, peak expiratory flow rate is noted at A. Peak inspiratory flow rate is noted at B. The lower portion of the loop represents inspiration and the upper portion, expiration. Flow-volume loops are plotted similarly to pulmonary function tests in which exhalation is plotted first followed by the next inspiration.

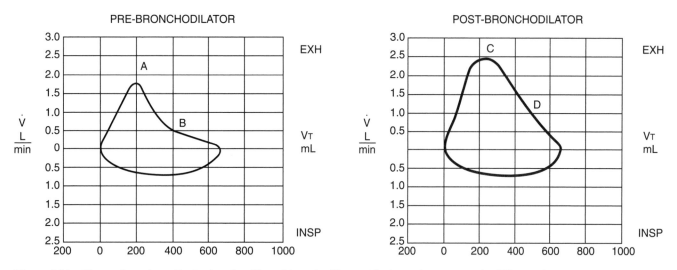

Figure 2.31 Flow-volume loop. Evaluating the effect of bronchodilators. The loops demonstrate the difference in peak expiratory flow rate, pre-, and post-bronchodilator therapy (A and C). In addition the scalloped shape near the end of exhalation (B) is characteristic of poor airway conductivity pre-bronchodilator, which is markedly improved with bronchodilators (D).

Period of Use	Recommendation	Rationale for Recommendation	Level of Recommendation	Supporting References	Comments
Selection of patients (continued)	Tracings can be saved for reference. Because changes in airway pressure occur slightly after changes in pleural pressure, there is a 0.2-second delay between hemodynamic changes and changes in airway pressure. Of note, agitation and rapid respiratory rates may make interpretation of hemodynamic measurements difficult (Figure 2.32).				

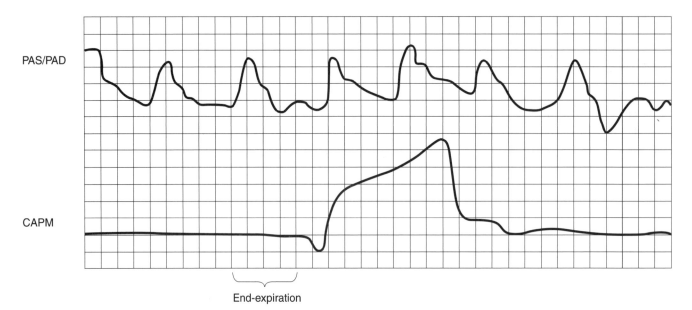

End-expiration

Figure 2.32   Tracing of pulmonary artery pressure combined with tracing of airway pressure. Airway pressure waveform shows end-expiration. Negative deflections indicate spontaneous effort by the patient. This patient was receiving intermittent mandatory ventilation. PAS = pulmonary artery systolic pressure; PAD = pulmonary artery diastolic pressure; CAPM = continuous airway pressure monitoring.

Period of Use	Recommendation	Rationale for Recommendation	Level of Recommendation	Supporting References	Comments
Selection of patients (continued)	**Monitoring of sponta-neous respiratory effort in patients receiving muscle relaxants**				
	A goal of neuromuscular blockade is to improve oxygenation and ventilation by controlling ineffi-cient breathing patterns caused by agitation or hyperdynamic states. Patients treated with neu-romuscular blockade may benefit from CAPM (ie, *pressure-time*), because it can be used to detect *breakthrough breathing*. A negative deflection indicating spontaneous effort (ie, *breakthrough)* is conclu-sive evidence that muscle relaxation is not com-plete. Use of CAPM is especially helpful when titrating the dosage of neuromuscular blocking agents. When used in this manner, CAPM will show the return of spon-taneous diaphragmatic effort before other neuro-logical signs become	In patients requiring neuro-muscular blockade, use of CAPM (eg, pressure-time monitoring) as a means of monitoring *breakthrough breathing* may eliminate the need for frequent peripheral nerve stimula-tion. However, CAPM *may not* be as sensitive an indi-cator of the level of block-ade when paralysis is attained. For continued neuromuscular blockade, peripheral nerve stimula-tion is a better indicator of drug requirements. Standard end-tidal CO_2 monitoring, which detects changes in flow, may be more sensitive than CAPM, which detects changes in pressure.	III: Laboratory data only, no clinical data to support recommendations II:	See Annotated Bibliography: 1, 2, 3, 6	

Period of Use	Recommendation	Rationale for Recommendation	Level of Recommendation	Supporting References	Comments
Selection of patients (continued)	apparent, enabling the clinician to intervene as necessary, before physiologic decompensation occurs (Figure 2.33).				
Application of device and initial monitoring	**Standard equipment** **Ventilator graphic respiratory waveform displays** No special equipment is required if the graphic display is part of the ventilator system. Follow the manufacturer's directions for specific waveform graphic displays. However, if the goal is to display the ventilator waveform graphics on the patient bedside monitor, a slave hard wire connection will be required to connect the ventilator waveform graphic displays to the bedside monitor. The reader is referred to the ventilator manufacturer's operating manual to determine how to accomplish this. The hospital engineering department may also need to be consulted. Use of CAPM requires that a channel of the bedside cardiac monitor be dedicated to monitoring pressure-time waveforms continuously. Additional components				

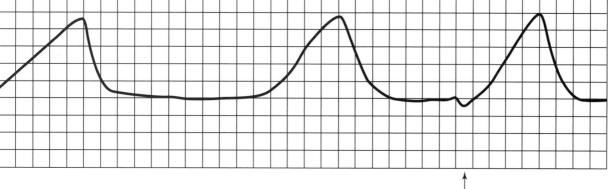

Figure 2.33 Breakthrough in a patient receiving a neuromuscular blocking agent and assist-control ventilation. Arrow at negative deflection indicates spontaneous diaphragmatic effort by the patient.

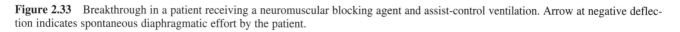

Period of Use	Recommendation	Rationale for Recommendation	Level of Recommendation	Supporting References	Comments
Application of device and initial monitoring (continued)	required are a transducer cable and high-pressure tubing, such as that used for monitoring PA and arterial pressures. **Setup for CAPM** Figure 2.34 shows the setup of a CAPM system. The steps are as follows: 1. Assemble the tubing and connect it to the transducer. 2. Because no fluid will be connected to the system, discard the infusion spike end of the tubing and cap the port. 3. Connect the distal end of the tubing to the ventilator circuit at the Y-connector. Any adapter that provides a tight connection can be used. Special connectors are manufactured specifically for CAPM, but other adapters can also be used. 4. Because the reference level is atmosphere (approximately 760 mm Hg, or sea level), zeroing is accurate at *any* level. The position of the patient does not affect the accuracy of the system. Calibrate the system in accordance with the monitoring system's standard procedure except as follows: do not prime the tubing with fluid (use air only), and be aware	A CAPM system does not require fluid because it is transmitting the pressures of gases in motion.			

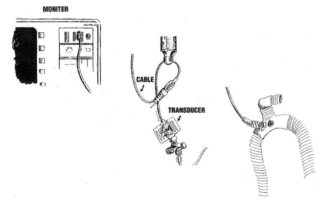

Figure 2.34   System for continuous airway pressure monitoring. Used with permission. Aloi A, Burns SM. Continuous airway pressure monitoring in the critical care setting. *Crit Care Nurse.* 1995;15(2):67.

Period of Use	Recommendation	Rationale for Recommendation	Level of Recommendation	Supporting References	Comments
Application of device and initial monitoring (continued)	that zeroing can occur at any level, because the reference level is atmosphere. 5. Place the waveform on the 0 to 30 scale (or whatever scale provides the best visualization of the waveform without interfering with other waveforms). 6. Graph the waveform as needed. The waveform will be displayed continuously.				
Ongoing monitoring	Respiratory waveform displays are helpful to determine changes in patient status. However, because the graphic displays are not usually integrated with other cardiac and hemodynamic parameters their use may be limited to periodic evaluation vs continuous monitoring. In contrast, because CAPM is integrated into the bedside monitor displays, observation of the pressure-time waveforms is easy to assess in conjunction with PA pressures and cardiac rhythms. CAPM can be used to check for disconnection and as a backup system for existing disconnect alarms. This feature is especially important in patients who require neuromuscular blockade. With some monitoring systems, the waveforms can be *floated* to different monitoring sites, thus providing an additional safeguard if a nurse must monitor more than 1 patient. The accuracy of the waveforms is obvious at a glance. Damping occurs with fluid in the tubing, such as secretions or condensation, and with leaks in the system. Thus, it is				

Period of Use	Recommendation	Rationale for Recommendation	Level of Recommendation	Supporting References	Comments
Ongoing monitoring (continued)	important to check connections for tightness and to clear the tubing if the waveform deteriorates. To clear the tubing, simply disconnect it and flush it with an air-filled syringe. Keep the Y-connector adapter in an upright position so the tubing is not gravity dependent and more likely to fill with fluid or secretions.				
	Zeroing should occur with initial application and with disconnections.				
	The type and frequency of documentation of respiratory waveforms and/or CAPM depend on the policy of the individual unit or institution and how they are used clinically (see the earlier section on competency).				
Device removal and quality control	To remove the CAPM system, disconnect it from the Y-connector and the monitor. Cap the Y-connector adapter to prevent a circuit leak.				
	In general, change the tubing with each change in ventilator circuitry (following the unit's routine) and as needed. Because the diameter of the tubing is small, problems with condensation may occur, requiring more frequent changes in the tubing.				
	If the waveform graphics are part of an integrated ventilator system, removal and quality control issues may vary. Refer to the product manufacturer's guidelines for specific information.				

ANNOTATED BIBLIOGRAPHY

1. **Aloi A, Burns SM. Continuous airway pressure monitoring in the critical care setting.** *Crit Care Nurse.* **1995;15(2):66–74.**

This article describes a clinical method of CAPM and delineates 3 clinical applications: continuous assessment of a patient's response to ventilator modes, accurate interpretation of hemodynamic measurements, and continuous visual monitoring of patients who are paralyzed because of chemically induced neuromuscular blockade. Numerous examples of waveforms and a step-by-step description of how the system is set up are included.

2. **Truwit JD, Rochester DF. Monitoring the respiratory system of the mechanically ventilated patient.** *New Horiz.* **1994;2:94–106.**

This clinical article describes numerous invasive and noninvasive monitoring methods for use in patients receiving mechanical ventilation. Specifically, the authors recommend monitoring airway pressure in all patients who require neuromuscular blockade. They note that this type of monitoring is a noninvasive means of achieving patient-ventilator synchrony without excessive degrees of muscle relaxation. Because airway pressure monitoring is used to detect diaphragmatic activity, neuromuscular blocking agents can be titrated accordingly.

3. **Truwit JD, Marini JJ. Evaluation of thoracic mechanics in the ventilated patient, part 1: primary measurements.** *J Crit Care.* **1988;3:133–150.**

This review focuses on techniques for assessing effort intensity, the pattern and rhythm of the breathing cycle, and the physical properties of the lung and chest wall during mechanical ventilation. The authors suggest that monitoring airway pressure be used to help detect signs of ventilatory distress and impending respiratory failure and to provide simple, accurate information on cycle timing. They also note the importance of using airway pressure monitoring to detect patient-ventilator asynchrony.

4. **Ahrens TS. Effects of mechanical ventilation on hemodynamic waveforms.** *Crit Care Nurs Clin North Am.* **1991;3:629–639.**

This article discusses the effects of positive-pressure ventilation on hemodynamic waveforms. It shows how to accurately detect end-expiration by monitoring airway pressure. Accurate detection of end-expiration is essential for the correct measurement of PA pressures, because both spontaneous (negative pressure) and mechanical (positive pressure) breaths distort PA waveforms. Although the article is not a research study, it is grounded in sound physiologic principles.

5. **Ahrens TS. Airway pressure measurement as an aid to identify end-expiration in hemodynamic waveform analysis.** *Crit Care Nurse.* **1992;12:44–48.**

This article by Ahrens is similar to the one published by the same author in *Critical Care Nursing Clinics of North America* in 1991 (see reference 4 in this list).

6. **Burns SM. Continuous airway pressure monitoring.** *Crit Care Nurse.* **2004;24:70–74.**

This is a review of continuous airway pressure monitoring and is derived from the AACN *Protocols for Practice* series on noninvasive monitoring. The article describes CAPM, applications, and setup.

7. **Puritan Bennett.** *Ventilator waveforms: graphical presentation of ventilatory data.* **Pleasanton, Calif: Nellcor Puritan Bennett Inc.; 2003.**

This helpful handbook describes the interpretation and potential application of pressure-time, flow-time, volume-time and loop configurations (pressure-volume and flow-volume).

8. **Burns SM. Working with respiratory waveforms: how to use bedside graphics.** *AACN Clin Issues: Adv Pract Acute Crit Care.* **2003;14(2):133–144.**

This article describes how to interpret respiratory waveforms and suggests clinical applications.

End-Tidal Carbon Dioxide Monitoring

Robert E. St. John, MSN, RN, RRT

CHAPTER THREE

End-Tidal Carbon Dioxide Monitoring

CASE STUDY

Mrs Thomas is a 63-year-old woman who was admitted to the hospital after 2 days of fever, shortness of breath, cough, and progressive muscle weakness. In the emergency department, respiratory failure developed, necessitating intubation and mechanical ventilation. During the next 48 hours, pneumococcal pneumonia was diagnosed, and appropriate antibiotic treatment was started. After 4 days of treatment and supportive care, the nursing, respiratory, and physician staff decided to try weaning Mrs Thomas from mechanical ventilation. As part of the overall evaluation, an end-tidal carbon dioxide monitor was set up to assess trends in ventilation. During the subsequent weaning, Mrs Thomas experienced a progressive increase in spontaneous respirations (20 to 36 breaths/minute), a decrease in spontaneous tidal volume (an average of 350 to 225 ml/breath). The end-tidal CO_2 level went from 36 to 32 mm Hg with an acceptable capnographic waveform. Pulse oximetry values were unchanged at 94% to 92%. Physical assessment by a nurse and analysis of arterial blood confirmed adequate oxygenation and a decrease in alveolar ventilation gases ($PaCO_2$ of 45), which was noted as a lower $PETCO_2$ reflective of an increase in dead-space ventilation and thus subsequently a lower $PETCO_2$. At this point, because of increased respiratory muscle work and possible fatigue, the nurse elected to terminate the weaning trial.

GENERAL DESCRIPTION

The end-tidal carbon dioxide monitor used for this patient consisted of a stand-alone electronic bedside noninvasive respiratory monitor that continuously measures exhaled carbon dioxide on a breath-by-breath basis. Depending on the type of equipment used, the concentration of inspired and expired carbon dioxide can be measured directly at the patient-ventilator circuit interface (mainstream sensor; **Figure 3.1**), or a sample of gases can be collected and transported via small-bore tubing to the bedside monitor (conventional or low-flow sidestream; **Figure 3.2**) for measurement.

Concentrations of respired carbon dioxide from the patient's airway are typically determined by using infrared light. With this method, the absorption of carbon dioxide molecules exposed to various wavelengths of light within a sample chamber or cell is measured. A photodetector then compares the relative amount of light absorbed by the sample with the amount absorbed by a gas that is free of carbon dioxide. The difference between the 2 represents the concentration of carbon dioxide. Another method used to analyze exhaled gases is mass spectrometry, which separates

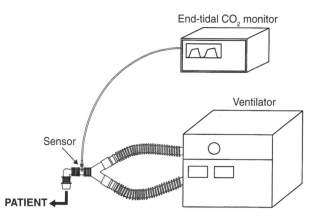

Figure 3.1 Mainstream end-tidal carbon dioxide monitor with measurement sensor and sample chamber at the patient-ventilator circuit interface.

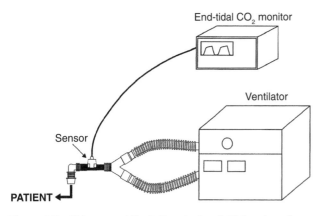

Figure 3.2 Sidestream (distal-diverting) end-tidal carbon dioxide monitor with the sampling port and the tubing that transports gas to the monitor for analysis.

and measures breath-by-breath respired gas on the basis of molecular weight. Because of the cost and labor required to maintain the sophisticated equipment required for mass spectrometry, infrared monitors are more commonplace outside the anesthesia environment.

A capnometer provides a visual analog or digital display of the concentration of exhaled carbon dioxide either as a percentage or as millimeters of mercury. In addition, most end-tidal carbon dioxide monitors also produce visual waveform recordings of the concentrations of inspired and exhaled carbon dioxide that can be examined either on a

breath-by-breath basis or for long-term trends. If these graphic displays are calibrated, the bedside instrument is called a capnograph.

The waveforms can usually be visualized at several speeds. In general, the fast-speed recordings provide a real-time display of the carbon dioxide waveform on a breath-by-breath basis. A normal fast-speed waveform or capnogram has a characteristic appearance that represents the various phases of carbon dioxide elimination in the lungs during exhalation (**Figure 3.3**). On the other hand, slow-speed capnograms show trends of carbon dioxide levels over various periods, from minutes to hours. In many clinical situations, capnograms can provide useful information about a patient's condition (**Figures 3.4 through 3.13**).

The ideal electronic bedside end-tidal carbon dioxide monitor provides both numeric and graphic waveform displays. The display on the monitor represents the highest concentration of carbon dioxide reached at the end of exhalation and is assumed to represent alveolar gas, which under normal ventilation-perfusion matching in the lungs closely parallels arterial levels of carbon dioxide. The normal arterial to end-tidal CO_2 gradient or difference ($PaCO_2$ - $P_{ET}CO_2$) is approximately 1 to 5 mm Hg.

In order to ensure accurate measurements during capnography with infrared light technology, most instruments incorporate various external and internal features that are designed to stabilize readings and minimize interference caused by either gas sampling and transport or the technique used for analysis. These components differ depending on the manufacturer and play an important role in the overall bias and precision ratings of each instrument.

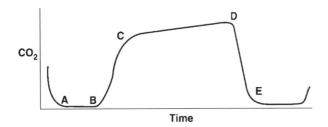

Figure 3.3 Typical normal carbon dioxide waveform. A to B, Exhalation of carbon dioxide-free gas from dead space. B to C, Combination of dead space and alveolar gases. C to D, Exhalation of mostly alveolar gas (alveolar plateau). D, End-tidal point, that, exhalation of carbon dioxide at maximum point. D to E, Inspiration begins and the carbon dioxide concentration rapidly falls to baseline or zero. (Reprinted by permission. Nellcor Puritan Bennett, a unit of Tyco Healthcare, Pleasanton, Calif.)

ACCURACY

Most electronic bedside capnographs can measure concentrations of CO_2 within a range of 0 to 100 mm Hg or 0% to 10%. The overall accuracy of measurement varies depending on the unit but typically is within ± 2 mm Hg for values between 0 and 40 mm Hg. Beyond this range, the accuracy of individual instruments varies more, in the range of ± 4 to ± 8 mm Hg, but clinicians should review the manufacturer's specifications for each instrument. Many authors suggest that the numeric display of the concentration of end-tidal carbon dioxide not be relied upon without visual examination of the capnographic

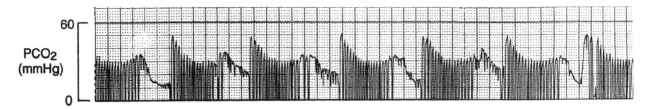

Figure 3.4 Slow-speed capnogram shows Cheyne-Stokes respirations in a 72-year-old woman who required mechanical ventilation after a cerebral vascular accident. Note the changes in breathing pattern associated with periods of apnea that consistently repeat.

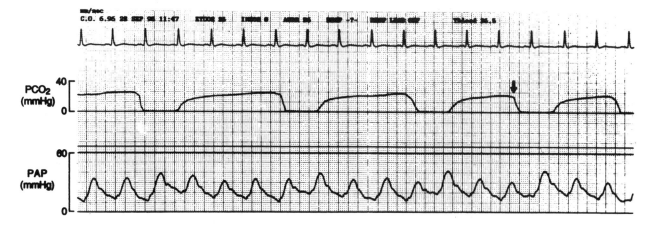

Figure 3.5 Real-time electrocardiogram, end-tidal carbon dioxide waveforms, and pulmonary artery pressures (PAPs) in a 43-year-old man after a cardiac arrest. Note the location of end-tidal carbon dioxide (arrow), which denotes end-expiration and also indicates the proper point at which to measure PAP.

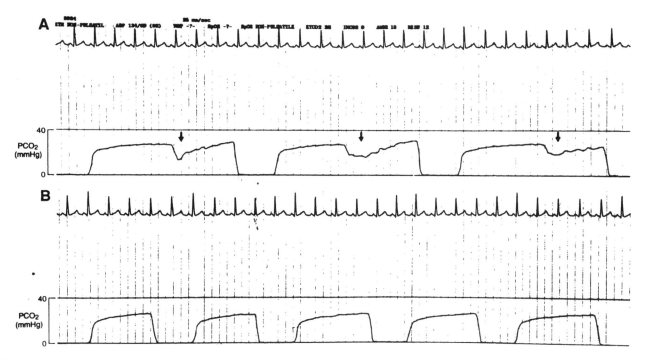

Figure 3.6 Electrocardiograms and capnograms of a 57-year-old man receiving mechanical ventilation for respiratory failure associated with bacterial pneumonia. A, Respiratory efforts (arrows) are not being sensed by the ventilator because the trigger sensitivity control is set inappropriately. B, Correction of the sensitivity setting allows the patient to trigger the ventilator on demand.

waveform as a quality indicator (see **Figures 3.4 through 3.13** for examples of abnormal waveforms).

Aside from technical considerations, the accuracy and reliability of end-tidal carbon dioxide monitors come under question clinically when the patient has abnormal changes in ventilation and perfusion. For the concentration of end-tidal carbon dioxide to reflect what is happening to the carbon dioxide level in arterial blood, pulmonary blood flow must be evenly matched with ventilation. When an uneven pattern occurs, such as when ventilation is greater than perfusion, the difference between $PaCO_2$ and $PETCO_2$ increases, sometimes

reaching a gradient of 20 mm Hg or higher. When this occurs, the $PETCO_2$ does not reflect $PaCO_2$. Therefore, because ventilation-perfusion matching in critically ill patients is often abnormal, $PETCO_2$ values displayed by the monitor must be evaluated cautiously. However, routine monitoring of the $PaCO_2$–$PETCO_2$ gradient may be valuable for determining trends. For example, a gradual narrowing of the gradient over time may represent improved ventilation-perfusion matching and pulmonary function.

It is also important to recognize that end-tidal carbon dioxide monitoring depends on adequate pulmonary blood flow to

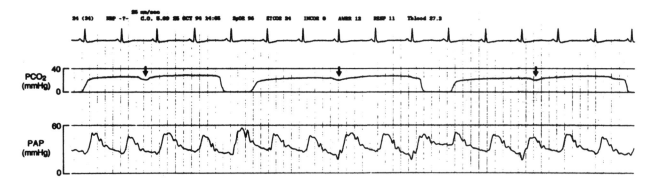

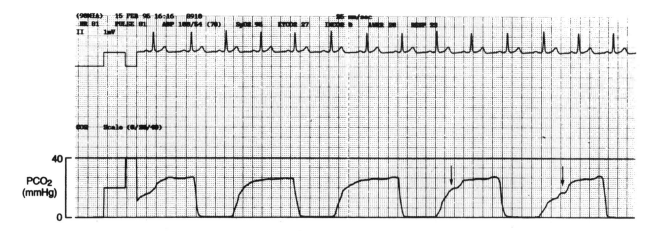

Figure 3.7   Real-time electrocardiogram, end-tidal carbon dioxide waveforms, and pulmonary artery pressures (PAPs) in a 67-year-old woman who was receiving mechanical ventilation because of respiratory distress and urosepsis. She was also receiving a sedative and a neuromuscular blocking agent. The end-tidal carbon dioxide waveforms show break-through spontaneous respiratory efforts (arrows) that are too weak to trigger a ventilator breath.

Figure 3.8   Electrocardiogram and capnogram of a 34-year-old man recovering from a drug overdose. The patient is orally intubated and occasionally bites the endotracheal tube (arrows), causing a partial obstruction to exhaled airflow.

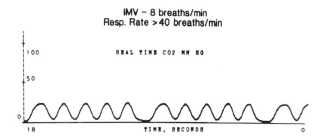

Figure 3.9   Elevated spontaneous respiratory rate during intermittent mandatory ventilation (IMV) obscures mechanical breaths, which can be detected only by a slightly longer pause after tidal exchange. Note unfavorable respiratory pattern, with no alveolar plateau and low $P_{ET}CO_2$. (With permission, Carlon GC et al. Capnography in mechanically ventilated patients. *Crit Care Med.* 1998;16(5):550–556.)

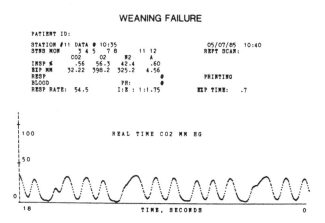

Figure 3.10   Chaotic respiratory pattern in a patient unable to tolerate spontaneous ventilation. (With permission, Carlon GC et al. Capnography in mechanically ventilated patients. *Crit Care Med.* 1998;16(5):550–556.)

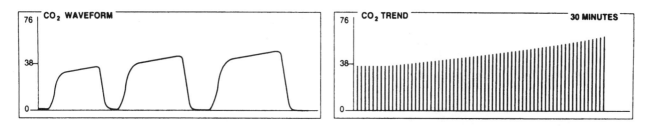

Figure 3.11 High-speed (left) and slow-speed (right) capnograms show an increasing PETCO$_2$. This pattern is associated with hypoventilation, increasing production of carbon dioxide, and absorption of carbon dioxide from an exogenous source such as carbon dioxide laparoscopy. An extremely rapid rise in PETCO$_2$ may suggest malignant hyperthermia. (Reprinted by permission, Nellcor Puritan Bennett, a unit of Tyco Healthcare, Pleasanton, Calif.)

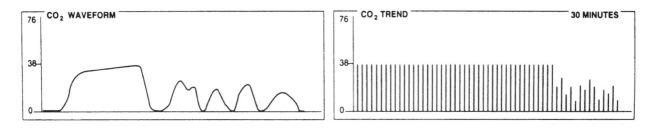

Figure 3.12 High-speed (left) and slow-speed (right) capnograms show a sudden drop of PETCO$_2$ to a low but nonzero value in incomplete sampling of a patient's exhalation. System leaks or partial airway obstruction may be present. (Reprinted by permission, Nellcor Puritan Bennett, a unit of Tyco Healthcare, Pleasanton, Calif.)

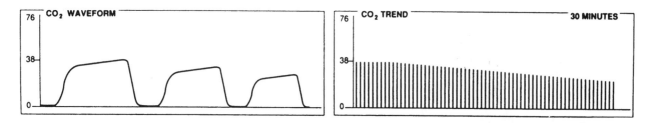

Figure 3.13 High-speed (left) and slow-speed (right) capnograms show a gradual decrease in PETCO$_2$. This pattern indicates decreasing production of carbon dioxide or decreasing pulmonary perfusion. (Reprinted by permission, Nellcor Puritan Bennett, a unit of Tyco Healthcare, Pleasanton, Calif.)

transport carbon dioxide to the lungs for elimination and subsequent measurement. For example, during cardiac arrest, there is no active pulmonary blood flow and therefore no carbon dioxide waveform. There is increasing laboratory and clinical evidence to suggest that end-tidal carbon dioxide monitoring may be a useful tool for evaluating the effectiveness of cardiopulmonary resuscitation aimed at reestablishing circulation.

Although end-tidal carbon dioxide monitoring is utilized most often in patients with artificial airways such as an endotracheal or tracheostomy tube, there is increasing experience with its use in nonintubated spontaneously breathing patients for various surgical or endoscopic procedures and procedural sedation (**Figure 3.14**). In fact, the American Society of Anesthesiologists state in the *Practice Guidelines for Sedation and Analgesia by Non-Anesthesiologists*, "Automated apnea monitoring (by detection of exhaled carbon dioxide or other means) may decrease risks during both moderate and deep sedation."

They emphasize that because ventilation and oxygenation are separate though related physiological processes, monitoring oxygenation by pulse oximeter is not a substitute for the monitoring of ventilatory function. They recommend that all patients undergoing sedation should be monitored by pulse oximetry and that monitoring exhaled carbon dioxide should be considered for all patients receiving deep sedation and also for those whose ventilation cannot be directly observed during moderate sedation. Further, the use of end-tidal carbon dioxide monitoring during pre-hospital transport offers a simple, effective method of monitoring respiratory status for intubated and nonintubated patients.

COMPETENCY

Effective use of end-tidal carbon dioxide monitoring requires knowledge of pulmonary anatomy and physiology,

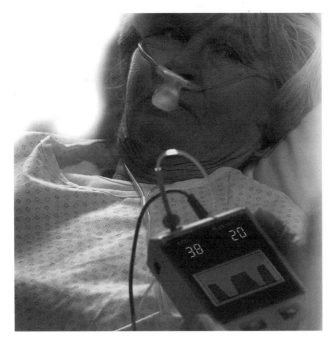

Figure 3.14   Bedside end-tidal dioxide monitoring using a nasal sampling technique and a hand-held portable capnography device. (Photo with permission, Oridion Capnography, Needham, Mass.)

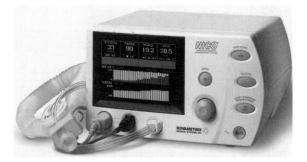

Figure 3.15   Noninvasive cardiac output monitor, which incorporates a partial carbon dioxide rebreathing method and end-tidal carbon dioxide measures in mechanically ventilated patients. (Photo with permission, Novametrix Medical Systems, Inc., Wallingford, Conn.)

knowledge of the procedures and purposes of end-tidal carbon dioxide monitoring, and analysis of arterial blood gases. Additionally, for verification of competency, nurses should demonstrate the ability to do the following:

- Set up the monitoring equipment, and perform a calibration check as recommended by the manufacturer.
- Assemble the monitoring circuit correctly and connect the monitor to the patient.
- Ensure that the circuit is functioning properly and that an accurate reading or waveform is obtained.
- Ensure that the monitoring equipment is functioning properly.

FUTURE RESEARCH

Although numerous clinical studies describe the advantages and limitations of using capnography to reflect changes in arterial levels of carbon dioxide, additional research is needed to identify new promising applications and to better define the patients for whom its use might be of benefit. The technology of end-tidal carbon dioxide monitoring has expanded to allow direct interface with many bedside physiologic monitoring systems. Continual cardiac output measurement using end-tidal carbon dioxide has been recently introduced. This technique uses a method known as partial CO_2 rebreathing, which is based on the well-established Fick principle. With this method, cardiac output is proportional to the change in CO_2 elimination divided by the change in $PETCO_2$ resulting from a brief rebreathing period.

A special monitor is commercially available (**Figure 3.15**), which allows for direct bedside measurement, and research is ongoing comparing this technique against traditional invasive thermodilution-based cardiac output using the pulmonary artery catheter. Another use of end-tidal carbon dioxide is in the calculation of volumetric carbon dioxide. Volumetric CO_2 is the integration of 2 well-established technologies, airway flow and mainstream capnography, which combine to form the volumetric CO_2 graph. The integration provides information such as CO_2 elimination (VCO_2), airway deadspace, and alveolar volume. Such information can be used for ventilator management, including monitoring and weaning. In addition, semiquantitative nonelectronic methods using chemically sensitive paper that changes color in the presence of carbon dioxide on a breath-to-breath basis are in widespread use for hospital, transport, and emergency medicine (**Figure 3.16**). Recently, this detection device has been used for verifying feeding tube placement, and further research in this area is needed.

Irrespective of quantitative measures of $PETCO_2$, the waveform display alone can often provide helpful information. It can be used to detect respiratory effort not easily determined by physical examination; abnormal respiratory breathing patterns, such as Cheyne-Stokes respirations; the response to adjustments in ventilator settings, such as positive end-expiratory pressure or tidal volume; ventilator malfunction or disconnection; and excessive air leaks around the artificial airway or ventilator circuitry. It can also be used to detect displacement of endotracheal tubes, verify placement of endotracheal tubes in the lung, and assess the level of paralysis induced with neuromuscular blocking agents. Although many of these advantages are well described in the literature on the use of capnographic waveforms during anesthesia, further research is needed in the critical care, emergency, and acute care settings to better determine the clinical usefulness of end-tidal carbon dioxide monitoring beyond the numerical display provided.

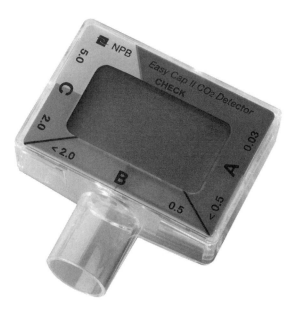

Figure 3.16 Example of a colorimetric carbon dioxide detector for use with manual resuscitation bags. (Photo with permission, Nellcor Puritan Bennett, a unit of Tyco Healthcare, Pleasanton, Calif.)

SUGGESTED READINGS

These resources provide additional information for those users who may wish to learn more about this technology.

Ahrens T, Sona C. Capnography application in acute and critical care. *AACN Clin Issues.* 2003;14:123–132.

Araujo-Preza CE, Melhado ME, Gutierrez FJ, et al. Use of capnometry to verify feeding tube placement. *Crit Care Med.* 2002;30:2255–2259.

Benumof JL. Interpretation of capnography. *AANA J.* 1998;66:169–176.

Burns SM, Carpenter R, Truwit JD. Report on the development of a procedure to prevent placement of feeding tubes into the lungs using end-tidal CO_2 measurements. *Crit Care Med.* 2001;29:936–939.

Carlon GD, Ray C, Miodownik S, Kopec I, Groeger JS. Capnography in mechanically ventilated patients. *Crit Care Med.* 1988;16:550–556.

Deakin CD, Sado DM, Coats TJ, et al. Prehospital end-tidal carbon dioxide concentration and outcome in major trauma. *J Trauma.* 2004;57:65–68.

Hess D. Capnometery and capnography: technical aspects, physiologic aspects, and clinical applications. *Respir Care.* 1990;35:557–573.

Kotake Y, Moriyama K, Innami Y, et al. Performance of noninvasive partial CO_2 rebreathing cardiac output and continuous thermodilution cardiac output in patients undergoing aortic reconstruction surgery. *Anesthesiology.* 2003;99:283–288.

Levine RL, Wayne MA, Miller CC. End-tidal carbon dioxide and outcome of out-of-hospital cardiac arrest. *N Engl J Med.* 1997;337:301–306.

McArthur CD. AARC clinical practice guideline. Capnography/capnometry during mechanical ventilation—2003 revision & update. *Respir Care.* 2003;48:534–539.

Miner JL, Heegard W, Plummer D. End-tidal carbon dioxide monitoring during procedural sedation. *Acad Emerg Med.* 2002;9:275–280.

Verschuren F, Liistro G, Coffeng R, et al. Volumetric capnography as a screening test for pulmonary embolus in the emergency department. *Chest.* 2004;125:841–850.

American Society of Anesthesiologists. *Practice Parameter: Practice Guidelines for Sedation and Analgesia by Non-Anesthesiologists.* Revised 2001.

CLINICAL RECOMMENDATIONS

The rating scales for the Level of Recommendation column range from I to VI, with levels indicated as follows: I, manufacturer's recommendation only; II, theory based, no research data to support recommendations, recommendations from expert consensus group may exist; III, laboratory data only, no clinical data to support recommendations; IV, limited clinical studies to support recommendations; V, clinical studies in more than 1 or 2 different populations and situations to support recommendations; VI, clinical studies in a variety of patient populations and situations to support recommendations.

Period of Use	Recommendation	Rationale for Recommendation	Level of Recommendation	Supporting References	Comments
Selection of Patients	No exclusion in adults on the basis of age or physical condition.				
	End-tidal carbon dioxide monitoring is typically used in intubated patients.	Detection of end-tidal carbon dioxide is best when all exhaled air passes through an airway adapter.	VI: Clinical studies in a variety of populations and situations	See Annotated Bibliography: 1, 2, 3–5, 8, 9	It is preferable in most patient situations that the monitor sample or measure from an artificial airway does not have any leak around the cuff. Some low-flow device systems are able to monitor reliably in the face of minor leaks so long as the volume needed for an adequate signal is present. Ideally, all exhaled air should pass through the airway adapter used to measure carbon dioxide.
	End-tidal carbon dioxide monitoring can also be used in non-intubated spontaneously breathing patients.	In patients who are not intubated, monitoring is done via a modified nasal cannula using either a conventional or low-flow sidestream capnometer. A mainstream configuration may be used with certain facemasks in nonintubated patients.	V: Clinical studies in more than 1 or 2 different patient populations and situations to support recommendations	See Other References: 2, 23, 26, 34–35	Clinical data on the use of end-tidal carbon dioxide monitoring in nonintubated patients is increasing due to advances in sampling technology. However, proper fit of the sampling cannula is critical in order to obtain reliable readings. Even so, the data suggest that $P_{ET}CO_2$ values determined in this manner may be variable and should be interpreted carefully. Values obtained may be helpful for assessing directional trends.
	Indications for use include the following: • Evaluating the efficacy of ventilation during mechanical ventilation	The concentration of end-tidal carbon dioxide normally reflects the concentration of alveolar carbon dioxide, which in turn reflects arterial carbon dioxide tension ($PaCO_2$) under conditions of normal ventilation and perfusion matching.	VI: Clinical studies in a variety of populations and situations	See Other References: 1, 4, 6, 8, 11–12, 37	

Period of Use	Recommendation	Rationale for Recommendation	Level of Recommendation	Supporting References	Comments
	• Monitoring ventilator circuit integrity and ventilator malfunction	Often, disruption of expired airflow caused by conditions such as loose tubing connections, circuit disconnection, obstruction, and machine malfunction can be detected by examining the capnogram.	VI: Clinical studies in a variety of populations and situations	See Other References: 10–13, 16, 24, 37	End-tidal carbon dioxide waveforms often provide qualitative information that a solitary quantitative $PETCO_2$ numerical reading does not.
Selection of Patients (*cont.*)	• Monitoring the effectiveness of cardiopulmonary resuscitation	The absence or presence of pulmonary blood flow during cardiopulmonary resuscitation can be reflected by changes in $PETCO_2$ levels.	V: Clinical studies in more than 1 or 2 different patient populations and situations to support recommendations	See Other References: 3, 31, 33, 45	The relationship between $PaCO_2$ and $PETCO_2$ is extremely variable, depending on the patient's clinical situation. Thus, although studies suggest that the overall correlation is satisfactory, the observed individual variation is such that unless ventilation-perfusion (V/Q) matching is normal, measuring $PETCO_2$ should not be used as a substitute for measuring $PaCO_2$ in all situations. Measurements of $PETCO_2$ used in conjunction with measurements of $PaCO_2$ may be useful for detecting acute changes in either alveolar ventilation or pulmonary blood flow. End-tidal carbon dioxide monitoring may also be useful for assessing and determining trends in the changes in a patient's condition over time that affect alveolar ventilation or pulmonary blood flow.
	• Monitoring during weaning from mechanical ventilation	If ventilation-perfusion matching is normal, $PETCO_2$ trends during weaning should reflect changes in alveolar ventilation.	VI: Clinical studies in a variety of populations and situations to support recommendations	See Other References: 1, 4, 12, 37–38	
	• Monitoring during intentional hyperventilation therapy used to control increased intracranial pressure	Measurement of $PETCO_2$ levels provides a rapid, noninvasive assessment of alveolar ventilation that might be useful when attempting to keep the $PETCO_2$ within a narrow range.	IV: Limited clinical studies to support recommendations	See Other References: 22, 41	
	• Monitoring as an adjunctive tool to screen for pulmonary embolism	Measurement of $PETCO_2$ levels may be helpful where pulmonary blood flow is suddenly reduced due to obstruction. Some have advocated volumetric capnography in conjunction with d-dimer.	IV: Limited clinical studies to support recommendations	See Other References: 36, 38	
	• Capnography can be incorporated in an alternative method for cardiac output determination by a modification of the cardiovascular Fick equation. Patient must be intubated.	In the partial carbon dioxide rebreathing method, monitored changes in CO_2 elimination and $PETCO_2$ response to a brief rebreathing period are used to estimate cardiac output.	IV: Limited clinical studies to support recommendations	See Other References: 25, 28–30	
	• Verifying correct placement of an endotracheal tube	So long as pulmonary blood flow is present, the detection of exhaled carbon dioxide with each breath will verify that the tube is in the lung.	VI: Clinical studies in a variety of populations and situations to support recommendations	See Other References: 39–40, 43–45	Both the American College of Emergency Physicians and international guidelines for emergency cardiovascular care recommend use of end-tidal carbon dioxide monitoring as a method for verifying endotracheal tube placement. (Colorimetric carbon dioxide detectors are adequate for this application.) Low cardiac output

(continued)

Period of Use	Recommendation	Rationale for Recommendation	Level of Recommendation	Supporting References	Comments
					may cause a false negative result when attempting to verify endotracheal tube placement. False positive results can occur with an endotracheal tube in the pharynx and when antacids and/or carbonated beverages are present in the stomach.
	• Detecting breathing effort during neuromuscular blockade	Measurement of $P_{ET}CO_2$ levels might be used in conjunction with peripheral nerve stimulation as a sensitive means of detecting patients' spontaneous respiratory efforts. These efforts are often referred to as a "curare cleft," which is visualized on the capnogram (Figure 7).	IV: Limited clinical studies to support recommendations	See Other References: 8–9, 37	
Selection of Patients (*cont.*)	• Confirmation of non-pulmonary nasogastric tube placement during insertion	The absence of carbon dioxide detection during insertion of the nasogastric tube is thought to indicate non-pulmonary or gastrointestinal placement.	V: Clinical studies in more than 1 or 2 different patient populations and situations to support recommendations.	See Other References: 16–21	Although capnometry monitors can be used for this purpose, there are several published reports of successful use of colorimetric carbon dioxide detectors (Easy Cap, Nellcor, Pleasanton Calif) attached to the end of the nasogastric tube.
	• Monitoring during procedural sedation	Safety monitoring of ventilatory status via $P_{ET}CO_2$ during administration of intravenous narcotics and sedatives is faster responding than oxygen desaturation as a result of hypoventilation.	VI: Clinical studies in a variety of populations and situations to support recommendations	See Other References: 2, 27, 35	Advances in monitoring technology now allow for reliable $P_{ET}CO_2$ measurement in nonintubated patients undergoing procedural sedation.
Application of Device and Initial Monitoring	End-tidal carbon dioxide monitors may require periodic calibration. Refer to the manufacturer's guidelines for specific information about calibration procedures.	Improper calibration may lead to erroneous $P_{ET}CO_2$ values.	I: Manufacturer's recommendation only	Product manufacturer's operating manual See Other References: 6, 7	All companies that manufacture end-tidal carbon dioxide monitors use some type of calibration procedure. The key benefit for clinicians is selecting a monitor that is easily and quickly calibrated.
	Do not accept $P_{ET}CO_2$ values without first determining the quality of the capnogram.	A poor quality $P_{ET}CO_2$ waveform will often display numeric values that are of questionable value.	VI: Clinical studies in a variety of populations and situations to support recommendations	See Other References: 1, 4, 11, 13, 37–38	
	Initially, correlate the $P_{ET}CO_2$ value with a carbon dioxide value obtained by arterial blood gas analysis of a blood sample obtained at the same time as the $P_{ET}CO_2$ value.	Confirmation of the correlation between arterial and end-tidal concentrations of carbon dioxide is helpful when establishing a value for determining trends in the changes in $PaCO_2$.			Breathing frequency may affect the capnograph by exceeding the response capabilities of certain monitors.

Period of Use	Recommendation	Rationale for Recommendation	Level of Recommendation	Supporting References	Comments
	Regardless of the type of the sampling technique, do the following:				
	• Place the airway adapter or sampling port as close as possible to the patient's airway. Position the airway adapter in an upright position according to the manufacturer's recommendations.	Obtaining samples of gas farther away from the patient will result in a delay in detecting changes in PETCO$_2$.			The closer the airway measuring adapter and sensor (mainstream) or sampling port (sidestream) are placed to the patient-ventilator connection, the more responsive the monitor will be when detecting a change in the level of exhaled carbon dioxide.
					If the airway adapter and sampling ports are not kept upright, water condensate and secretions will pool at the bottom of the adapter and may interfere in the measurement of carbon dioxide. Use of filters between the patient's airway and the sampling line may lead to erroneous PETCO$_2$ readings.
Application of Device and Initial Monitoring (*cont.*)	• Support the positioning of the airway adapter or sampling port to minimize pull or weight on the patient's airway.	Excessive pull or weight could displace the endotracheal tube and cause discomfort to the patient.			
	• Determine alarm settings for respiratory rate, apnea default, high and low PETCO$_2$ levels, and minimum levels of inspiratory carbon dioxide according to the policy of the institution or the physician's order.	As a surveillance system for detecting either immediate changes or trends over time, default alarm settings for values outside the normal range are important. The absolute alarm set point should be individualized for each patient.			Depending on the monitor, high and low alarm settings can usually be set by the clinician. It is important to adjust the limits so that alarms will activate before too drastic a change occurs in the patient's condition.
					The normal PaCO$_2$ – PETCO$_2$ difference or gradient is 1 to 5 mm Hg. In disease states that affect ventilation-perfusion matching in the lung, this gradient may increase significantly to 20 mm Hg or more. Conditions that increase dead-space ventilation (ie, high V/Q) will result in wider PaCO$_2$ – PETCO$_2$ gradients. This difference should be documented when the device is initially set up and used thereafter for determining trend.

Period of Use	Recommendation	Rationale for Recommendation	Level of Recommendation	Supporting References	Comments
Ongoing Monitoring	Initially, set the monitor to display continuous numeric PETCO$_2$ values as well as waveforms on a breath-by-breath basis. In some instances, using slow-speed recordings over a specific interval to determine trends may be appropriate.	The numerical display of the PETCO$_2$ should not be accepted without first determining the quality of the PETCO$_2$ waveform.	VI: Clinical studies in a variety of populations and situations to support recommendations	See Annotated Bibliography: 6, 7 See Other References: 8–10	

COMMENTS

The PETCO$_2$ waveform is most commonly displayed in a fast-speed mode (25 mm/sec) to provide detailed graphic waveforms for each exhaled breath on a continuous basis. The appearance of the waveform not only helps confirm the acceptability of the numerical PETCO$_2$ displayed but may also be helpful for detecting rapid changes in a patient's condition, such as air leak, airway obstruction, sudden loss in carbon dioxide reading, suggesting extubation or displacement of an endotracheal tube outside the lung, or acute loss of pulmonary blood flow. Fast-speed capnograms, aside from the numerical value, may also be used in conjunction with monitoring of pulmonary artery pressure to detect the point of end-expiration in tachypneic patients or during nontraditional modes of ventilation, such as inverse-ratio ventilation. Waveform monitoring on a breath-by-breath basis may also be useful in detecting respiratory effort by the patient; ventilator synchrony and asynchrony; and in some cases, malfunction of ventilator equipment that would not be easily detected by clinical observation alone.

The waveforms can also be displayed or recorded at a slow speed (12.5 mm/sec or slower) for determining trends. This slow speed may be particularly helpful in detecting changes in a patient's condition that occur over fixed periods such as minutes or hours. For example, slow-speed trends of each individual PETCO$_2$ waveform could be used to detect changes in breathing pattern, such as Cheyne-Stokes respirations or to determine the interval between occurrence and discovery of a progressive endotracheal cuff leak.

Period of Use	Recommendation	Rationale for Recommendation	Level of Recommendation	Supporting References	Comments
Device Removal	Dispose of airway adapters or sampling ports and tubing designed for 1-time use after use in a patient or if they become obstructed and interfere with proper detection of carbon dioxide levels.	Disposable adapters and ports are often made of material that cannot be cleaned between patients for extended use. Follow the manufacturer's guidelines for cleaning procedures and solutions to use when the adapters and ports are in use.	I: Manufacturer's recommendation only	Product manufacturer's operating manual	
	Clean reusable cables, modules, and bedside monitors between patient use according to the manufacturer's recommendations.	Patients' risk of infection increases when proper cleaning procedures are not followed. Cleaning solutions and sterilizing methods that are not approved by the manufacturer may damage the equipment.			Improperly processed reusable equipment is a potential source of pathogens. Although the potential may vary, airway adapters that will come in contact with the patient's lungs should be disinfected by using the most effective high-level method available, according to the manufacturer's recommendations.
	Clean reusable cables, modules, and bedside monitors between patient use according to the manufacturer's recommendations.	Reusable components should be cleaned to prevent the spread of infection.			Cables and monitoring components that either are not in contact with the patient or touch only intact skin have low potential for infection and may only require low- or intermediate-level disinfection. It is best to follow the manufacturer's suggestions to avoid damage to the equipment.

Period of Use	Recommendation	Rationale for Recommendation	Level of Recommendation	Supporting References	Comments
Prevention of Complications	Steps to prevent complications include the following: **ALL END-TIDAL CARBON DIOXIDE MONITORS**				
	After the initial calibration, do subsequent recalibration checks according to the manufacturer's recommendations.	Most manufacturers suggest that periodic calibration checks be done while the monitor is in operation. Checking the system for zero carbon dioxide as well as with a fixed or known level of carbon dioxide tests the linearity of the measuring sensor.	I: Manufacturer's recommendation only	Product manufacturer's operating manual See Other References: 11–14	Although most end-tidal carbon dioxide monitoring systems have internal components or features that stabilize readings, periodic checks of calibration while the monitor is in use may be recommended to ensure readings are technically correct. Follow the manufacturer's guidelines at a minimum, but realize that the system can be checked more often if the technical accuracy of the monitor may be a problem.
	Maintain the position of the airway sensor or sample port close to the artificial airway (endotracheal tube).	Moving the sampling or measuring site farther away from the patient-ventilator interface reduces the monitor's ability to provide a sharp and rapid response to changes in $PETCO_2$.			
	MAINSTREAM MONITORS Keep the sample measurement window or chamber in the airway clear of secretions.	Blockage of infrared light in the sample measurement chamber will interfere with detection of carbon dioxide.	I: Manufacturer's recommendation only		Whenever verifying a displayed $PETCO_2$ reading by comparing it with a $PaCO_2$ measurement, it is important to document the $PETCO_2$ reading as the arterial blood is being drawn for analysis, not before or afterward.
	If the measuring sensor generates a significant amount of heat, take steps to prevent the sensor from contacting the patient's skin. A heat shield or other protective device can be used.	Excessive heat associated with certain capnometers can cause thermal injury to tissue if direct skin contact occurs.			All monitors, depending on the design, have certain routine operating requirements that must be maintained for correct sampling and measuring of exhaled air. It is critical to adhere strictly to the manufacturer's recommendations for sampling tubing, cable use, positioning of the adapters, and so forth. Never mix gas-sampling or measuring equipment from a manufacturer with that from another unless the compatibility of the equipment is specified in writing. Damage to the equipment and injury to the patient might occur.
	Observe for degree of weight and pull on the artificial airway by the addition of the sampling airway adapter and measurement sensor.	Excessive pull on the artificial airway by some airway adapters or sensors can cause changes in the position of an endotracheal tube or discomfort to the patient.			

Period of Use	Recommendation	Rationale for Recommendation	Level of Recommendation	Supporting References	Comments
Prevention of Complications (*cont.*)	SIDESTREAM MONITORS Position the sample port so that it is not contaminated with ambient air.	The expired airstream at the patient connection is the optimal sampling site for proper measurement. If leaks or loose connections occur, ambient air may contaminate the measured sample, resulting in falsely low $PetCO_2$ readings.	I: Manufacturer's recommendation only		
	Use of nafion tubing may be acceptable, depending on the manufacturer.	Using sampling tubing of the proper type, size, and length ensures safe and accurate measurement of $PetCO_2$.			
	Use water traps or filters as required by the manufacturer.	Failure to follow the manufacturer's guidelines may result in damage to the equipment and possible injury to the patient.			
	Be sure the tubing used for sampling is impermeable to carbon dioxide and leak free.				
	If using a modified nasal cannula tubing designed for end-tidal carbon dioxide monitoring in nonintubated patients, ensure that device is sized properly in order to optimize carbon dioxide sampling for measurement.	Always follow manufacturer's guidelines when using the dedicated nasal cannula sampling tubing for monitoring.	I: Manufacturer's recommendation only		Improper positioning will lead to falsely low $PetCO_2$ readings.
	NOTE: When using a mass spectrometer instrument for end-tidal carbon dioxide monitoring, exercise caution when taking $PetCO_2$ readings during activation of the meter dose inhaler in the breathing circuit.	The presence of freon as a propellant in meter dose inhalers can result in falsely high $PetCO_2$ readings.			
Quality Control Issues	If required by the manufacturer, check the calibration of the monitor daily or more often while the equipment is in clinical use.	Periodic calibration checks are necessary to ensure properly functioning equipment.		Product manufacturer's operating manual	Follow the same suggestions given for quality control measures to ensure accurate and reliable readings.
	Inspect the capnogram before accepting the numerical $PetCO_2$ readout.	Poor-quality waveforms may indicate technical problems with $PetCO_2$ measurement.		See Other References: 11, 13, 15	

Period of Use	Recommendation	Rationale for Recommendation	Level of Recommendation	Supporting References	Comments
Quality Control Issues (*cont.*)	Inspect airway adapters and ports for air leakage and obstructions at least once each nursing shift.	Loose connections may cause air leaks, resulting in loss in tidal volume delivery and falsely low $PetCO_2$ readings. Obstruction of the sampling tubing (sidestream) or the measurement window in the airway adapter (mainstream) will cause errors in measurement.			
	Whenever the numerical $PetCO_2$ reading is questionable and the waveform is acceptable, obtain an arterial blood gas analysis for confirmation of possible changes in the $PaCO_2$.	With proper sampling technique, noninvasive measures such as $PetCO_2$ reflect $PaCO_2$ only under conditions of normal ventilation-perfusion matching.	VI: Clinical studies in a variety of patient populations and situations	See Other References: 1, 4, 6–7, 10, 12, 38	It is important to recognize that $PETCO_2$ is not the same as $PaCO_2$. In theory, the $PETCO_2$ reflects the partial pressure of alveolar carbon dioxide ($PaCO_2$). The $PaCO_2$ results from the overall degree of ventilation-perfusion matching in the lungs. If the ventilation-perfusion ratio is normal, then $PETCO_2$ will approximate the arterial carbon dioxide tension or $PaCO_2$.

As mentioned previously, the difference or gradient between $PaCO_2$ and $PETCO_2$ is normally small (1 to 5 mm Hg). It is possible, however, for the $PETCO_2$ to be higher than the $PaCO_2$. The physiologic reasons for this are not well understood but may be related to regions of low ventilation-perfusion matching within the lung. |

ANNOTATED BIBLIOGRAPHY

1. **Hess D, Schlottag A, Levin B, Mathai J, Rexode W. An evaluation of the usefulness of end-tidal P_{CO_2} to aid weaning from mechanical ventilation following cardiac surgery.** *Respir Care.* **1991;36:837–843.**

Study Sample

Twenty-four patients, 41 to 74 years old, who were intubated and receiving mechanical ventilation after cardiac surgery.

Comparison Studied

The purpose of the study was to determine if changes in $P_{ET}CO_2$ could be used as an indication of changes in $PaCO_2$ during postoperative weaning from mechanical ventilation.

Study Procedures

$P_{ET}CO_2$ was monitored continuously during weaning from mechanical ventilation. The number of comparisons of $PaCO_2$ and $P_{ET}CO_2$ per patient ranged from 3 to 9. The $P_{ET}CO_2$ values used for comparison were obtained at the time of routine drawing of blood for analysis of arterial blood gases.

Key Results

Overall correlations between single-point comparisons of $PaCO_2$ and $P_{ET}CO_2$ were acceptable. The ability of $P_{ET}CO_2$ to precisely indicate changes in $PaCO_2$ was limited. The mean difference between $PaCO_2$ and $P_{ET}CO_2$ was 4.0 ± 3.7 mm Hg (range, -5 to 16 mm Hg). In 38 (43%) of 89 instances in which changes in $P_{ET}CO_2$ were compared with changes in $PaCO_2$, the $P_{ET}CO_2$ value incorrectly indicated the direction of change in $PaCO_2$. For changes in P_{CO_2} greater than or equal to 5 mm Hg, $P_{ET}CO_2$ incorrectly indicated the change in direction of $PaCO_2$ in 14 (30%) of 46 comparisons.

Study Strengths and Weaknesses

The strengths of the study include the specific population examined, the good descriptions of the methods used, and the relatively large number of observations (n = 113). In addition, capnographic waveforms were inspected for all measurements, multiple comparisons were done for each patient, and comparisons were made for more than 1 mode of ventilation. The weaknesses are the limited ability to generalize findings to other populations of patients and not using the same number of paired comparisons for each patient.

Clinical Implications

The results of the study suggest that $P_{ET}CO_2$ values should not be used alone to reflect changes in $PaCO_2$. The authors recommend further studies in other populations to evaluate the role of noninvasive monitoring, clinical skills, and analysis of arterial blood gases during weaning from mechanical ventilation.

2. **Yamanaka M, Sue D. Comparison of arterial-end-tidal P_{CO_2} difference and dead space/tidal volume ratio in respiratory failure.** *Chest.* **1987;92:832–835.**

Study Sample

Seventeen patients, 25 to 80 years old, in a medical-respiratory ICU who required mechanical ventilation.

Comparison Studied

$PaCO_2$ vs $P_{ET}CO_2$ and the arterial to end-tidal carbon dioxide gradient vs dead space (V_D/V_T).

Study Procedures

Measurements on each patient were completed within a 20-minute period. The accepted $P_{ET}CO_2$ value represented a 30-second average. Values of V_D/V_T were determined by analysis of samples of mixed expired gases, and an estimated CO_2 output value was used in the V_D/V_T calculation.

Key Results

The investigators found large differences between $PaCO_2$ and $P_{ET}CO_2$ in individual patients. The $PaCO_2 - P_{ET}CO_2$ gradient varied from 0 to 39 mm Hg and correlated closely with V_D/V_T ($r = 0.80$, $p < .05$).

Study Strengths and Weaknesses

A strength of the study is that the subjects are representative of patients typically seen in a medical-respiratory ICU. In addition, the measurements of V_D/V_T were technically done well. The weaknesses include the small sample size, the lack of multiple measurements on each patient, use of only 1 mode of ventilation (assist control), and limited statistical analysis. Although the type and model number of the end-tidal carbon dioxide monitor are given, calibration and validation of the technical accuracy and reliability of the monitor are not described.

Clinical Implications

The authors conclude that in their study population of nonsurgical patients, $PaCO_2$ cannot be reliably estimated on the basis of $P_{ET}CO_2$ and that measurements of $P_{ET}CO_2$ should not be used as a substitute for measurements of $PaCO_2$. They theorize that this lack of reliability is due to changes in ventilation and perfusion distribution that occur in patients with pulmonary disease. They suggest that the efficiency of ventilation can be indicated by the difference between $P_{ET}CO_2$ and $PaCO_2$. The difference can be used as an estimate of wasted or dead space ventilation.

3. **Levine RL, Wayne MA, Miller CC. End-tidal carbon dioxide and outcome of out-of-hospital cardiac arrest.** *N Engl J Med.* **1997;337:301–306.**

Study Sample

The study sample consisted of 150 consecutive victims of cardiac arrest outside the hospital who had electrical activity but no pulse.

Comparison Studied

The prospective study sought to determine whether death could be predicted by monitoring end-tidal carbon dioxide during resuscitation after cardiac arrest.

Study Procedures

For each cardiac arrest, patients were intubated and evaluated by mainstream capnography. Paramedics followed standard advanced-cardiac life support protocols with on-line medical control from a single base station. $PETCO_2$ was monitored continuously and recorded on a form attached to the patient's emergency services record.

Key Results

A total of 150 patients were included in the data analysis. There was no difference in the mean age or initial $PETCO_2$ between patients who survived to hospital admission (survivors) and those who did not (nonsurvivors). After 20 minutes of advanced cardiac life support measures, $PETCO_2$ averaged 4.4 ± 2.9 mm Hg in the nonsurvivors and 32.8 ± 7.4 mm Hg in the survivors ($p = .001$). A 20-minute end-tidal carbon dioxide value of 10 mm Hg or less successfully discriminated between the 35 patients who survived to hospital admission and the 115 nonsurvivors. When a 20-minute $PETCO_2$ value of 10 mm Hg or less was used as a screening test to predict death, the sensitivity, specificity, positive predictive value, and negative predictive value were all 100%. The authors conclude that when the $PETCO_2$ is 10 mm Hg or less measured 20 minutes after the initiation of advanced cardiac life support, resuscitation efforts may reasonably be terminated.

Study Strengths and Weaknesses

The study population was well defined, using a clinically relevant condition of cardiac arrest involving electrical activity without a pulse. Capnography was initiated early (at the beginning of resuscitation efforts) and the entire study was performed outside the hospital, without introducing variables such as transportation to a new environment. The study cannot be used to determine which of the patients in whom spontaneous circulation is restored will be long-term survivors. Other dysrhythmias and patient populations need to be studied before the study conclusions can be extended to other patients with cardiac arrest. Lastly, patients presenting with significant ventilation-perfusion abnormalities such as obstructive lung disease or pulmonary emboli may have lower than normal baseline $PETCO_2$ levels, and may mask response to treatment aimed at improving survival.

Clinical Implications

The authors conclude that $PETCO_2$ monitoring during resuscitation efforts can be a useful predictor of death from cardiac arrest in patients with electrical activity but no pulse. Measuring $PETCO_2$ is technically feasible outside the hospital. In this population, an end-tidal carbon dioxide level of 10 mm Hg or less measured after 20 minutes after the start of advanced cardiac life support accurately predicts death.

4. Burns SM, Carpenter R, Truwit JD. Report on the development of a procedure to prevent placement of feeding tubes into the lungs using end-tidal CO₂ measurements. *Crit Care Med.* 2001;29:936–939.

Study Sample

Twenty-five adult mechanically ventilated medical intensive care unit patients; 5 in phase 1 and 20 in phase 2 of the study.

Comparison Studied

The 2-phase study was designed to determine the accuracy of a technique using capnography to prevent inadvertent placement of small-bore feeding tubes and Salem sump tubes into the lungs.

Study Procedures

Phase 1 tested the ability of the end-tidal carbon dioxide ($PETCO_2$) monitor to detect flow through the small-bore feeding tubes. A small-bore feeding tube, with stylet in place, was placed 5 cm through the top of the tracheostomy tube ventilator adapter in 5 consecutive patients. The distal end of the feeding tube was attached to the capnography instrument. The $PETCO_2$ level and waveform were assessed and recorded. Because $PETCO_2$ waveforms were successfully detected, a convenience sample of 20 adult patients (Phase 2) who were having either small-bore feeding tube (n = 7) or Salem sump (n = 13) were studied. The technique consisted of attaching the $PETCO_2$ monitor to the tubes and observing for the capnographic waveform throughout placement.

Key Results

Of the 7 small-bore feeding tubes tested, all were successfully placed on initial insertion. Placement was confirmed by absence of a $PETCO_2$ waveform and by radiographic assessment. Of the 13 Salem sump tubes, 9 were placed successfully on the first attempt and confirmed by the absence of CO_2 and by manual syringe air bolus and aspiration of stomach contents. $PETCO_2$ waveforms were detected with insertion of 4 of the Salem sump tubes; the tubes were immediately withdrawn, and placement was reattempted until successful.

Study Strengths and Weaknesses

The article describes a simple, cost effective method of assuring accurate gastric tube placement in critically ill patients. Because the information is immediately available at the bedside using the monitor and is easy to interpret, this method would be relatively simple to implement. The study did not test nonintubated/nonventilated patients. In those situations where low spontaneous tidal volume breaths are present, the described method may not work as well without some modifications to the technique. These would represent areas of future potential study. The study size was relatively small and perhaps additional limitations might be discovered with the technique and procedure's reliability.

Clinical Implications

The authors conclude that continuous measurement of $PETCO_2$ during orogastric or nasogastric tube placement is easily performed and accurately identifies inadvertent placement into the lungs. The implementation of quality measures to prevent complications is a goal of institutions across the country. This preliminary study describes a promising technique, which may be considered for clinical application in acutely ill patient populations.

5. Miner JR, Weegaard W, Plummer D. End-tidal carbon dioxide monitoring during procedural sedation. *Acad Emerg Med.* 2002;9:275–280.

Study Sample

Seventy-four adult patients admitted to the emergency department undergoing procedural sedation were enrolled in the study.

Comparison Studied

The researchers studied the utility of $PETCO_2$ monitors to detect respiratory depression in patients undergoing procedural sedation. They also sought to determine whether the depth of sedation as perceived by the clinician can be predicted by the amount of respiratory depression detected by $PETCO_2$.

Study Procedures

This prospective, observational study involved obtaining baseline measures of vital signs, pulse oximetry, and $PETCO_2$ on each subject. The sedative agent(s) were recorded as well as pretreatment supplemental oxygen. During the procedure, pulse oximetry, blood pressure, heart rate, $PETCO_2$ and respiratory rate were recorded every 2 minutes, in addition to recording the nadir. The treating clinician also recorded the Observer's Assessment of Alertness/Sedation Scale (OAA/S) every 2 minutes during the procedure. Respiratory depression was defined as an oxygen saturation of <90% for at least 1 minute, and $PETCO_2$ > 50 mm Hg at any time, or airway obstruction with cessation of gas exchange at any time (noted by absent $PETCO_2$ waveform). The need for and duration of assisted ventilation was also noted.

Key Results

Of the 74 patients enrolled, 40 (54.1%) received methohexital, 21 (28.4%) received propofol, 10 (13.5%) received fentanyl and midazolam, and 3 (4.1%) received etomidate. Respiratory depression was seen in 33 (44.6%) patients. No correlation was detected between OAA/S and $PETCO_2$. Eleven (14.9%) patients required assisted ventilation at some point during the procedure. Post-hoc analysis revealed that all patients with respiratory depression had $PETCO_2$ > 50 mm Hg, an absent waveform, or an absolute change from baseline $PETCO_2$ > 10 mm Hg. Pulse oximetry detected respiratory depression in 11 of the 33 patients.

Study Strengths and Weaknesses

The strengths of the study include the prospective study design, obtaining baseline hemodynamic measures along with pulse oximetry and capnography as well as throughout the procedural sedation period. Weaknesses are the relatively small sample size, and because the study was observational in nature, there were no controls making it difficult to generalize the study conclusions about the differences in respiratory depression rates of the various agents used. Additional questions that the study did not address include whether hypoventilation, as evidenced by an elevated $PETCO_2$ by the monitor, is an indication that the patient is adequately sedated for a procedure. Further, would adding $PETCO_2$ monitoring result in fewer complications and does pulse oximetry add anything further to monitoring if $PETCO_2$ is being monitored and the patient's ventilatory status is known?

Clinical Implications

The authors conclude that using a measurement of $PETCO_2$ does not appear to predict the level of sedation in patients undergoing emergency department procedural sedation. When the criteria of an $PETCO_2$ > 50 mm Hg, an absolute change >10 mm Hg, or an absent waveform were applied, all respiratory depression was identified, regardless of the oxygen saturation. $PETCO_2$ monitoring may be a useful adjunct assessment tool during procedural sedation in detecting alveolar hypoventilation, allowing for early intervention.

6. Carlon GC, Ray C, Miodownik S, Kopec I, Groeger JS. Capnography in mechanically ventilated patients. *Crit Care Med.* 1988;16:550–556.

Description

This was not a formal research study. The authors compiled numerous examples showing the clinical use and benefit of capnographic waveforms in routine practice. They describe how these tracings can be used in the management of patients receiving mechanical ventilation. The paper describes cases in which capnographic waveforms were used to recognize technical failures not easily detectable by other means. The discussions and explanations of changes in waveforms due to therapeutic interventions are well grounded in pulmonary physiology theory.

7. Ahrens T, Sona C. Capnography application in acute and critical care. *AACN Clin Issues.* 2003;14:123–132.

Description

This is an excellent review article on capnography. The authors discuss the theoretic basis for end-tidal carbon dioxide monitoring and provide detailed information on the clinical application of this technique. Although this article does not represent a research study, it provides many examples of incorporating $P_{ET}CO_2$ values and waveform tracings as part of clinical management.

8. Thrush DN, Mentis SW, Downs JB. Weaning with end-tidal CO_2 and pulse oximetry. *J Clin Anesth.* 1991;3:456–460.

Study Sample

The study sample consisted of 10 adult patients (mean age 63 years) who were intubated and receiving mechanical ventilation after elective coronary artery bypass grafting. Excluded from the study were patients who had left ventricular and pulmonary dysfunction or who required valve replacement.

Comparison Studied

The study compared measurements of $P_{ET}CO_2$ and $PaCO_2$ obtained during postoperative weaning from mechanical ventilation. It also compared calculated SaO_2 values with SpO_2 values obtained by pulse oximetry during the weaning period.

Study Procedures

In this prospective study, $P_{ET}CO_2$ and SpO_2 were monitored continuously during reductions in ventilator rate.

Key Results

A total of 60 measurements were obtained. For all patients, a significant correlation was found between $PaCO_2$ and $P_{ET}CO_2$ ($r = 0.76$). The sensitivity of $P_{ET}CO_2$ for detecting hypercarbia was 95%. In 3 instances, hypercarbia ($PaCO_2$, >45 mm Hg) occurred when the $P_{ET}CO_2$ was less than 40 mm Hg. Overall, as the patient's ventilator rate was decreased, a significant decrease in the $PaCO_2$–$P_{ET}CO_2$ gradient occurred ($p < .001$)

Study Strengths and Weaknesses

The strengths of the study include its prospective study design and obtaining multiple measurements on each patient during reduction in ventilator rate (average, 6 per patient). Also, the end-tidal carbon dioxide monitor used in the study allowed assessment of capnographic waveforms. Weaknesses include the small sample size and the limited ability to generalize the findings to other populations of patients. Although the type and model number of the end-tidal carbon dioxide monitor are reported, the authors do not describe the methods used to ensure verification of proper waveforms or those used to calibrate and validate the technical accuracy and reliability of the monitor.

Clinical Implications

On the basis of their results, the authors conclude that continuous, noninvasive monitoring of SpO_2 and $P_{ET}CO_2$ is a reliable means of assessing patients during weaning from mechanical ventilation after coronary artery bypass grafting when adjustment of minute ventilation compensates for an increased $PaCO_2$–$P_{ET}CO_2$ gradient during controlled ventilation. The authors note that a potential disadvantage of weaning patients without using analysis of arterial blood gases could be unrecognized metabolic acidosis. Therefore, although they cannot advocate total abandonment of arterial blood gas analysis for postoperative patients, such analysis should rarely be necessary for safe and efficient weaning from mechanical ventilation after uncomplicated coronary artery bypass grafting in patients without significant left ventricular or pulmonary dysfunction.

OTHER REFERENCES

1. Hess D. Capnometry and capnography: technical aspects, physiologic aspects, and clinical applications. *Respir Care.* 1990;35:557–573.
2. Barton CW. Correlation of end-tidal CO_2 measurements to arterial $PaCO_2$ in nonintubated patients. *Ann Emerg Med.* 1994;23:562–563.
3. Falk JL, Rackow EC, Weil MH. End-tidal carbon dioxide concentration during cardiopulmonary resuscitation. *N Engl J Med.* 1988;318:607–611.
4. Task Force on Guidelines. Guidelines for standards of care for patients with acute respiratory failure on mechanical ventilatory support. *Crit Care Med.* 1991;19:275–285.
5. *Policy Statement on Expired Carbon Dioxide Monitoring.* Washington, DC: American College of Emergency Physicians; 1994.
6. Williamson JA, Webb RK, Cockings J, Morgan C. The capnograph: applications and limitations—an analysis of 2000 incident reports. *Anaesth Intensive Care.* 1993;21:551–557.
7. Raemer DB, Calalang I. Accuracy of end-tidal carbon dioxide analyzers. *J Clin Monit.* 1991;7:195–208.
8. Swedlow DB. Capnometry and capnography: the anaesthesia disaster early warning system. *Semin Anesth.* 1986;5:194–205.

9. Snyder JV, Elliot JL, Grenvik A. Capnography. In: Spence AA, ed. *Respiratory Monitoring in Intensive Care*. New York, NY: Churchill Livingstone; 1982: 100–121.

10. Stock MC. Noninvasive carbon dioxide monitoring. *Crit Care Clin*. 1988;4:511–526.

11. Schena J, Thompson J, Crone RK. Mechanical influences on the capnogram. *Crit Care Med*. 1984;12: 672–674.

12. Weingarten M. Respiratory monitoring of carbon dioxide and oxygen: a ten-year experience. *J Clin Monit*. 1990;6:217–225.

13. Zupan J, Martin M, Benumof JL. End-tidal CO_2 excretion waveform and error with gas sampling line leak. *Anesth Analg*. 1988;67:579–581.

14. Elliot WR, Raemer DB, Goldman DB, Philip JH. The effects of bronchodilator-inhaler aerosol propellants on respiratory gas monitors. *J Clin Monit*. 1991;7: 175–180.

15. Moorthy SS, Losasso AM, Wilcox J. End-tidal Pco_2 greater than $PaCO_2$. *Crit Care Med*. 1984;12:534–535.

16. Asai T, Stacy M. Confirmation of feeding tube position: how about capnography? *Anaesthesia*. 1994;49:451.

17. D'Souza C, Kilam SA, D'Souza U, et al. Pulmonary complications of feeding tubes: a new technique of insertion and monitoring malposition. *Can J Surg*. 1994;37:404–408.

18. Burns SM, Carpenter R, Truwitt JD. Report on development of a procedure to prevent placement of feeding tubes into the lungs using end-tidal CO_2 measurements. *Crit Care Med*. 2001;29:936–939.

19. Thomas BW, Falcone RE. Confirmation of nasogastric tube placement by colorimetric indicator detection of carbon dioxide. *J Am Coll Nurs*. 1998;17:195–197.

20. Kindopp AS, Drover JW, Heyland DK. Capnography confirms correct feeding tube placement in intensive care unit patients. *Can J Anaesth*. 2001;48:705–710.

21. Araujo-Preza CE, Melhado ME, Gutierrez FJ, et al. Use of capnometry to verify feeding tube placement. *Crit Care Med*. 2002;30:2255–2259.

22. Helm M, Schuster R, Hauke J, et al. Tight control of prehospital ventilation by capnography in major trauma victims. *Br J Anaesth*. 2003;90:327–332.

23. Casati A, Gallioli G, Scandroglio M, et al. Accuracy of end-tidal carbon dioxide monitoring using the NPB75 microstream capnometer. A study in intubated ventilated and spontaneously breathing nonintubated patients. *Eur J Anaesthesiol*. 2000;17:622–626.

24. Benumof JL. Interpretation of capnography. *AANA J*. 1998;66:169–176.

25. Binder JC, Parkin WG. Noninvasive cardiac output determination: comparison of a new partial rebreathing technique with thermodilution. *Anaesth Intensive Care*. 2001;29:19–23.

26. Casati A, Gallioli G, Passaretta R, et al. End tidal carbon dioxide monitoring in spontaneously breathing nonintubated patients. A clinical comparison between conventional sidestream and mircostream capnometers. *Minerva Anaesthesiol*. 2001;67:161–164.

27. Vargo JJ, Zuccaro G Jr, Dumot JA, et al. Automated graphic assessment of respiratory activity is superior to pulse oximetry and visual assessment for the detection of early respiratory depression during therapeutic upper endoscopy. *Gastrointest Endosc*. 2002;55:826–831.

28. Jopling MW. Noninvasive cardiac output determination utilizing the method of partial CO_2 rebreathing. A comparison with continuous and bolus thermodilution cardiac output. *Anesthesiology*. 1998;89:(3a), A544.

29. Gama de Abreu M, Quintal M, Ragaller M, et al. Partial carbon dioxide rebreathing: a reliable technique for noninvasive measurement of nonshunted pulmonary capillary blood flow. *Crit Care Med*. 1997;25:675–683.

30. Kotake Y, Moriyama K, Innami Y, et al. Performance of noninvasive partial CO_2 rebreathing cardiac output and continuous thermodilution cardiac output in patients undergoing aortic reconstruction. *Anesthesiology*. 2003;99:283–288.

31. Deakin CD, Sado DM, Coats TJ, et al. Prehospital end-tidal carbon dioxide concentration and outcome in major trauma. *J Trauma*. 2004;57:65–68.

32. Ahrens T, Schallom L, Bettorf K, et al. End-tidal carbon dioxide measurements as a prognostic indicator of outcome in cardiac arrest. *Am J Crit Care*. 2001;10: 391–398.

33. Levine RL, Wayne MA, Miller CC. End-tidal carbon dioxide and outcome of out-of-hospital cardiac arrest. *N Engl J Med*. 1997;31:301–306.

34. Miner JR, Heegard W, Plummer D. End-tidal carbon dioxide monitoring during procedural sedation. *Acad Emerg Med*. 2002;9:275–280.

35. Sandlin D. Capnography for nonintubated patients: the wave of the future for routine monitoring of procedural sedation. *J Perianesth Nurs*. 2002;17:277–281.

36. Verschuren F, Liistro G, Coffeng R, et al. Volumetric capnography as a screening test for pulmonary emboli in the emergency department. *Chest*. 2004;125:841–850.

37. Ahrens T, Sona C. Capnography application in acute and critical care. *AACN Clin Issues*. 2003;14:123–132.

38. McArthur CD; AARC. AARC clinical practice guideline. Capnography/capnometry during mechanical ventilation. *Respir Care*. 2003;48:534–539.

39. Grmec S, Mally S. Prehospital determination of tracheal tube placement in severe head injury. *Emerg Med J*. 2004;21:518–520.

40. DeBoer S, Seaver M, Arndt K. Verification of endotracheal tube placement: a comparison of confirmation techniques and devices. *J Emerg Nurs*. 2003;29:444–450.

41. Kerr ME, Zempsky J, Sereika S, et al. Relationship between arterial carbon dioxide and end-tidal carbon dioxide in mechanically ventilated adults with severe head trauma. *Crit Care Med.* 1996;24:785–790.

42. Hardman JG, Mahajan RP, Curran J. The influence of breathing system filters on paediatric capnography. *Paediatr Anaesth.* 1999;9:35–38.

43. Sum Ping ST, Mehta MP, Symreng T. Reliability of capnography in identifying esophageal intubation with carbonated beverage or antacid in the stomach. *Anesth Analg.* 1991;73.

44. American College of Emergency Physicians. Clinical Policies Committee. Verification of endotracheal tube placement. *Ann Emerg Med.* 2002;40:551–552.

45. Guidelines 2000 for Cardiopulmonary resuscitation and emergency cardiovascular care: international consensus on science. *Circulation.* 2000;102:11–1370.

Noninvasive Blood Pressure Monitoring

Karen K. Giuliano, RN, PhD, FAAN

Noninvasive Blood Pressure Monitoring

CASE STUDY

Ms Johnson, a 52-year-old woman, was admitted to the chest pain center of the emergency department (ED) for evaluation because of recurrent episodes of chest pain. She is obese and has been using diuretics for hypertension for the past 3 years. Ms Johnson has been pain free and in sinus rhythm since admission to the ED. Her vital signs are being monitored every 30 minutes using a noninvasive blood pressure (NIBP) monitor with a *regular* adult-sized cuff because a large adult-sized cuff cannot be found. She is also lying flat on a stretcher with her NIBP arm hanging off the side of the stretcher. Her systolic pressure has ranged from 180 to 210 mm Hg, her diastolic pressure has ranged from 82 to 94 mm Hg, and her heart rate has been in the mid-80s. Two inches of nitroglycerin ointment have been applied for treatment of her hypertension until the oral anti-hypertensives take effect. Two hours after admission, the alarm on the NIBP monitor goes off and begins flashing. The display indicates a blood pressure of 150/78 mm Hg and a pulse rate of 60 beats per minute. According to the cardiac monitor, Ms Johnson is having frequent premature ventricular contractions and occasional bigeminy. An auscultated blood pressure using a large adult-sized cuff measures her blood pressure at 120/60 mm Hg. The NIBP monitor is disconnected and sent to the biomedical department to be checked. The accompanying note says that the machine is not working correctly and is indicating erroneously high pressures.

GENERAL DESCRIPTION

Since 1962, when the first NIBP monitor was made available for hospital use, clinicians have deliberated over the accuracy and reliability of automated NIBP devices. Most of these devices use the oscillometric method for determining mean arterial blood pressure (MAP), systolic blood pressure (SBP), and diastolic blood pressure (DBP). Oscillometric devices use a special blood pressure cuff that can detect oscillations or movement in the arterial walls created by cardiac contractions. These oscillations are transmitted by the cuff hose to a microprocessor within the monitor that uses cuff pressure information and oscillation amplitudes to determine blood pressure. It is *essential* that a properly sized cuff be used so that accurate blood pressures can be determined when using either an automated or ausculatory method of blood pressure measurement. A cuff that is too small will cause a falsely high blood pressure measurement, and a cuff that is too large will cause falsely low blood pressure measurements.

Generally speaking, with oscillometric devices, SBP is determined at the point when oscillations of the arterial wall increase rapidly and DBP at the point when the oscillations decrease rapidly as the cuff pressure decreases during deflation of the cuff. Most oscillometric NIBP monitors need more than 1 oscillation and a fairly regular pattern to determine where SBP and DBP occur during cuff deflation. A regular rhythm produces consistent oscillations in the arterial wall (measured as oscillation amplitudes by the NIBP monitor) that enable the monitor to determine where SBP and DBP occur. Oscillometric NIBP monitors have difficulty determining SBP and DBP in patients with irregular heart rhythms and frequent dysrhythmias, because no oscillation amplitudes are the same. Because MAP can be determined on the basis of single oscillation amplitude, the largest oscillation amplitude that occurs at the lowest cuff pressure, MAP is generally the parameter most accurately determined by NIBP devices. In this case study, Ms Johnson likely received unnecessary treatment for her hypertension because the cuff used was too small and led to erroneously high blood pressure readings.

Position of the arm and blood pressure cuff relative to the heart is also important. The arm should be placed at the level of the patient's heart for accurate blood pressure measurement. In this case, Ms Johnson's arm was hanging off the side of the stretcher, which likely further exacerbated the falsely high blood pressure reading displayed by the NIBP monitor.

PRECISION AND ACCURACY

The blood pressure determinations obtained with automatic NIBP devices come under question especially when the values are compared with those determined by direct measurements of arterial blood pressures. For example, indirect measurements of brachial arterial pressure obtained either manually using auscultation or with an NIBP monitor are often compared with measurements of radial arterial pressure using direct arterial cannulation.

As monitoring devices move from the central part of the body to more peripheral areas, normal physiology causes the systolic pressure peak to increase and the diastolic pressure trough to decrease. This normal physiologic difference makes it difficult to compare either systolic or diastolic blood pressure measurements taken in the same patient at different anatomical measurement sites. Differences in the obtained blood pressure measurements may be based on physiology rather than actual changes in the patient's hemodynamics. In fact, there can be a difference of up to 25 mm Hg between the centrally measured SBP and one measured at the radial artery. However, MAP remains relatively constant when measured at different sites throughout the arterial circuit. Since the MAP stays relatively consistent, comparisons from different sites can be made with much greater accuracy.

In addition, the use of MAP also makes it possible for a more accurate comparison between a direct invasive blood pressure measurement and an indirect noninvasive blood pressure measurement.

The clinical studies reviewed in the annotated bibliography demonstrated varying results with regard to which blood pressure (SBP, DBP, or MAP) varied the least from blood pressure measurements obtained invasively.

There are many additional factors that can alter the accuracy of the oscillometric blood pressure measurement (Table 4.1). For accurate determination of blood pressure, these factors must be recognized and minimized if automatic NIBP monitoring is to be used.

Some studies have shown that the average difference between blood pressures (SBP, DBP, and MAP) determined with various NIBP monitors and arterial pressures measured directly are approximately 5 mm Hg. They have also shown that occasionally the value of 1 determination obtained with

TABLE 4.1   Factors that decrease the accuracy of oscillometric blood pressure measurement

Cuff application	Cuff too loose
	Air in cuff before application
	Kinked or loose connection
Anatomy and physiology	PVCs
	Respiratory variation
	Calcified arteries
	Thoracic outlet syndrome
	Conically shaped arms
	Patient talking during measurement
Intrinsic movement	Shivering
	Seizures
	Arm motion
Extrinsic movement	External cuff compression
	Passive arm motion
	Active arm motion

Adapted from: Bridges EJ, Middleton R. Direct vs oscillometric monitoring of blood pressure: Stop comparing and pick one (A decision-making algorithm). *Crit Care Nurse.* 1997;17(3):58–72.

an NIBP monitor can vary as much as 37 mm Hg from the value obtained by invasive measuring. This pattern of variability underscores the importance of never basing treatment on a single NIBP determination without validating the accuracy of the measured value. In addition, most authors suggest that direct monitoring of arterial blood pressure should be used to titrate vasoactive drugs, because determination of blood pressure with NIBP devices can take several minutes.

The Association for the Advancement of Medical Instrumentation (AAMI) has established standards for the validation of automatic blood pressure monitoring. These limits are a mean difference of ± 5 mm Hg and a standard deviation of no more than 8 mm Hg when the automated device is compared to an auscultatory reference. All NIBP devices used should conform to this accepted standard.

COMPETENCY

Validation of competency in using an NIBP device should be done during an employee's initial orientation to ensure that the employee can do the following:

1. Set up the NIBP system, measure arm circumference at an appropriate place, and apply an appropriately sized NIBP cuff to the patient's extremity.
2. Place the extremity being used for BP measurement at the level of the heart.
3. Make sure all equipment being used for measurement is working properly.
4. Recognize and monitor for potential complications resulting from use of the NIBP system.

FUTURE RESEARCH

In critical and acute care, patients experiencing irregular heart rates and rhythms are common, and it would be useful to know more about the performance of NIBP monitors in this patient group. A few clinical studies have included patients with irregular heart rhythms and have reported that the NIBP monitor can be used to determine blood pressure in some of these patients but not in others. Therefore, they are not reliable in patients with irregular heart rates. Larger numbers of patients with irregular heart rates and rhythms need to be studied clinically to determine if blood pressure in this population can be measured reliably by NIBP monitors. In general, manufacturers do not claim that oscillometric devices are accurate when cardiac rhythms are irregular. However, future NIBP devices should include enhanced algorithms that can account for irregular heart rates and rhythms, since these are common physiologic occurrences in critically ill patients.

Another area of future research includes device performance comparisons between some of the different NIBP devices currently on the market. There are numerous NIBP manufacturers and very little current information on the measurement accuracy between any of these devices. Newer NIBP technologies that use arterial tonometry, radial artery compression/decompression, rate of pressure change, and photoelectric measurement of blood pressure are undergoing clinical study. These techniques are being promoted as alternatives to continuous invasive monitoring. However, published, peer-reviewed literature is scarce on these newer technologies. Thus it is yet unclear if they may be used reliably to determine blood pressure as quickly and as accurately as invasive methods.

SUGGESTED READINGS

The following suggested readings provide additional information about methods of blood pressure measurement for those users who wish to learn more about this technology. They are organized by content.

Direct and indirect methods of blood pressure monitoring

McGee BH, Bridges EJ. Monitoring arterial blood pressure: what you may not know. *Crit Care Nurse.* 2002;2(2):60–79.

Bridges EJ, Middleton R. Direct vs oscillometric monitoring of blood pressure: stop comparing and pick one (a decision-making algorithm). *Crit Care Nurse.* 1997;17(3):58–72.

Perloff D, Grim C, Flack J, et al. Human blood pressure determination by sphygmomanometry. *Circulation.* 1993; 88(5):2460–2470.

Larrivee C, Joseph DH. Strategies for teaching decision making: discrepancies in cuff versus invasive blood pressures. *Dimens Crit Care Nurs.* 1992;11(5):278–285.

Jones D, Appel L, Sheps S, Roccella E, Ledant C. Measuring blood pressure accurately: new and persistent challenges. *JAMA.* 2003;289(8):1027–1030.

Bur A, Herker H, Vlcek M, et al. Factors influencing the accuracy of oscillometric blood pressure measurement in critically ill patients. *Crit Care Med.* 2003;31(3):793–799.

Bur A, Hirschl M, Herkner H, et al. Accuracy of oscillometric blood pressure measurement according to the relation between cuff size and upper-arm circumference in critically ill patients. *Crit Care Med.* 2000;28(2):371–376.

Hemingway TJ, Guss DA, Abdelnur D. Arm position and blood pressure measurement. *Ann Intern Med.* 2004; 140(1):74–75.

Knowledge level of clinical practitioners in the routine measurement of blood pressure

McGhee BH, Woods SL. Critical care nurses' knowledge of arterial blood pressure monitoring. *Am J Crit Care.* 2001; 10(1):43–51.

Torrance C, Serginson E. Student nurses' knowledge in relation to blood pressure measurement by sphygmomanometry and auscultation. *Nurse Educ Today.* 1996; 16(6):397–402.

Edmonds ZV, Mower WR, Lovato LM, Lomeli R. The reliability of vital signs measurements. *Ann Emerg Med.* 2002;39(3):233–237.

Armstrong RS. Nurses' knowledge of error in blood pressure measurement technique. *Int J Nurs Pract.* 2002;8(3): 118–126.

Newer methods of blood pressure measurement currently being investigated

Belani K, Ozaki M, Hynson J, et al. A new non-invasive method to measure blood pressure: Results of a multicenter trial. *Anesthesiology.* 1999;91(3):686–692.

Philippe ED, Hebert JL, Coirault C. A comparison between systolic aortic root pressure and finger blood pressure. *Chest.* 1998;113(6):1466–1474.

Lehmann ED. Estimation of central aortic pressure aveform by mathematical transformation of radial tonometry pressure data. *Circulation.* 1998;98(2):186–187.

Hirschl MM, Binder M, Herkner H, et al. Accuracy and reliability of noninvasive continuous finger blood pressure measurement in critically ill patients. *Crit Care Med.* 1996;24(10):1684–1689.

Brinton TJ, Cotter B, Kailasam MT, et al. Development and validation of a noninvasive method to determine arterial pressure and vascular compliance. *Am J Cardiol.* 1997;80(3):323–330.

CLINICAL RECOMMENDATIONS

The rating scales for the Level of Recommendation column range from I to VI, with levels indicated as follows: I, manufacturer's recommendation only; II, theory based, no research data to support recommendations, recommendations from expert consensus group may exist; III, laboratory data only, no clinical data to support recommendations; IV, limited clinical studies to support recommendations; V, clinical studies in more than 1 or 2 different populations and situations to support recommendations; VI, clinical studies in a variety of patient populations and situations to support recommendations.

Period of Use	Recommendation	Rationale for Recommendation	Level of Recommendation	Supporting References	Comments
Selection of Patients	No exclusion based on age.	With appropriately sized cuffs and tubing, NIBP monitors can be used on patients of all ages.	VI: Clinical studies in a variety of populations and situations	Product manufacturer's operating manual	The accuracy of blood pressure determinations by NIBP monitors in patients with irregular heart rates and rhythms has been variable.
	A longer and wider cuff is necessary for obese patients or patients with large, muscular arms.	Proper cuff fit is one of the most important aspects of accurate blood pressure measurement.		See Other References: 1, 2, 4, 8	
	Do **not** use NIBP in patients with the following:			See Annotated Bibliography: 1–9	For infants, it may be preferable to use the palpatory or flush methods because of their inability to cooperate.
	• Highly irregular or rapid cardiac rhythms	Beat-to-beat variation of 15% or more can lead to prolonged, erroneous, or no detection of blood pressure by oscillometric devices.			In elderly patients with sclerotic vessels, systolic pressure may be overestimated.
	• Excessive bodily movement (shivering, seizures, restlessness) or excessive external movement (helicopter, ambulance transport, rapid-cycling ventilator)	Excessive movement of the patient's limbs or external movement can mimic the oscillations or movement detected by the NIBP cuff and lead to inaccurate readings.			Examples of NIBP performance ranges for measurements in adults are as follows:
	• Extreme hypotension or hypertension	NIBP monitors have performance limits; in rare circumstances they cannot determine extremes in blood pressure.			• SBP, 30–245 mm Hg • DBP, 10–210 mm Hg • MAP, 10–225 mm Hg
	Do not place an NIBP cuff on the following:				
	• The same extremity with an IV infusion line	Inflation of the cuff will impede IV flow.			
	• The same extremity where SpO_2 is being monitored	Inflation of the cuff can interfere with continuous pulse oximetry measurements, depending on the oximeter.			
	• An extremity with impaired circulation	NIBP monitors can inflate to high pressures and further compromise circulation to the extremity.			

Period of Use	Recommendation	Rationale for Recommendation	Level of Recommendation	Supporting References	Comments
Application of Device and Initial Monitoring	The upper arm is the preferred site for cuff placement.	The upper arm is at approximately the same horizontal plane as the heart (the reference point for zero pressure). It is also the preferred site in patients with low blood pressure or those in shock because peripheral vasoconstriction may make it difficult to determine pressure at more distal peripheral sites.	VI: Clinical studies in a variety of populations and situations	See Other References: 1, 2, 3, 4, 8 See Annotated Bibliography: 1–9	No matter what position the patient is in, be sure to place the site for blood pressure measurement at the level of the heart.
	The forearm and ankle can also be used.	The forearm and calf can be used when the upper arm cannot be used or for the patient's comfort. Studies have demonstrated the accuracy of pressures obtained with cuffs on the calf.		Product manufacturer's operating manual	Determination of blood pressure at the ankle can be a useful indication of blood flow in conditions in which blood flow in the lower extremity may be compromised (e.g., aortic dissection, aortic compression in pregnancy and labor), during intra-aortic balloon pumping, and for evaluation of peripheral vascular disease.
	Select the proper cuff size. Cuff width should equal 40% of arm circumference (Table 4.2). If a large adult-sized cuff does not fit the upper arm, place the cuff at a alternative site (forearm or calf).	A cuff that is too small will lead to falsely high readings and a cuff that is too large will lead to falsely low readings.			
	Expel all residual air in the cuff.	A cuff with residual air can lead to too loose a fit and inaccurate readings.			

TABLE 4.2   American Heart Association Recommended Bladder Dimensions for Blood Pressure Cuffs According to Arm Circumference[* 2]

Cuff	Bladder Width (cm)	Bladder Length (cm)	Arm Circumference Range at Midpoint (cm)
Newborn	3	6	<6
Infant	5	15	6–15[**]
Child	8	21	16–21[**]
Small Adult	10	24	22–26
Adult	13	30	27–34
Large Adult	16	38	35–44
Adult Thigh	20	42	45–52

[*]There is some overlap of the recommended range for arm circumference in order to limit the number of cuff sizes; use larger cuff when available.

[**]To approximate the bladder width/arm circumference ratio of 0.40 more closely in infants and children, additional cuffs are available.

Period of Use	Recommendation	Rationale for Recommendation	Level of Recommendation	Supporting References	Comments
Application of Device and Initial Monitoring (*cont.*)	Check the system for leaks.	Leaky systems can lead to inaccurate readings.			
	Make sure patients back is supported and legs are not dangling.	Falsely high readings may result.			
	Start operation of the monitor and set preferred alarm limits according to manufacturer's directions.	NIBP monitors vary by manufacturer in operation and setup.	VI: Clinical studies in a variety of populations and situations	See Other References: 1, 2, 3, 4, 8 See Annotated Bibliography: 1–9 Product manufacturer's operating manual	**Whenever there is any question about an NIBP determination, check the patient's status first.** If the blood pressure determination suggests an error in reading, repeat the NIBP or measure blood pressure using another method. Oscillometric blood pressure devices are not interchangeable.
	Compare initial NIBP determination with a recent measurement obtained with auscultation on the same arm.	Individual determinations by NIBP monitors can vary greatly for a single reading and should be compared with other data to verify accuracy.			
	If NIBP determinations do not correlate with comparison measurements, send the device for calibration.	NIBP monitors require calibration at regular intervals according to manufacturer recommendations.			Calibration of NIBP monitors at regular intervals may be recommended. Refer to the product manufacturer's operating manual for specific information on calibration.
Ongoing Monitoring	Most NIBP monitors can be programmed to operate in either a manual or an automatic mode. Manual modes require the operator to cue the machine for NIBP determinations.		VI: Clinical studies in a variety of populations and situations	Product manufacturer's operating manual See Annotated Bibliography: 2 See Other References: 1, 2, 3, 4, 8	To date, studies have not been done to compare the accuracy of blood pressures determined with rapid or *stat* NIBP monitoring with those determined by invasive measurement of arterial pressure.
	For automatic mode, the clinician is able to select the time interval to meet the clinical requirements of the patient.				In general, a 5-minute period between inflations of the NIBP cuff is recommended to avoid venous congestion.
	Some monitors are capable of monitoring blood pressure in a *stat* mode. This very rapid mode should be used in emergent situations only and for short periods.	The more frequent the NIBP determinations, the greater is the likelihood that venous congestion and tissue damage will occur. This is especially true with stat mode, because the cuff never completely deflates between determinations during this mode of operation. If frequent or continuous determinations are required, direct arterial monitoring should be considered.			

Period of Use	Recommendation	Rationale for Recommendation	Level of Recommendation	Supporting References	Comments
Ongoing Monitoring (*cont.*)	NIBP monitors may not give accurate measurements if the patient is in shock or has very low blood pressure.	In shock states, oscillations of the arterial wall can be too minimal for detection by an NIBP monitor.			
Device Removal	Cuffs designed for single use should be disposed of after use or if they become soiled.	Disposable cuffs are *not* intended for use on more than 1 patient.	I: Manufacturer's recommendation only	Product manufacturer's operating manual	
	Wash nondisposable cuffs between patients.	Soiled cuffs can be a medium for bacterial growth and possible contamination of the patient. Follow manufacturer's recommendations for cleaning the cuffs between use.	I: Manufacturer's recommendation only	Product manufacturer's operating manual	
	If the NIBP system is equipped with a battery, keep the monitor plugged in when the system is not in use.	Keeping the monitor plugged in allows time for the battery to be recharged.			
Prevention of Complications	If blood pressure is being monitored continuously, change the cuff site every 4 hours if making more than 2 determinations per hour. Otherwise, change the cuff site daily.	Petechiae and skin irritation can develop from skin compression. NIBP monitors can inflate to pressures of 350 mm Hg and can stay inflated for up to 2 minutes.	IV: Limited clinical studies to support recommendations I: Manufacturer's recommendation only	See Other References: 1, 2, 3, 4, 8	Studies have not been done to determine if a thin layer of cloth or gauze between the skin and the cuff *significantly* alters the readings of an NIBP monitor. However, if a patient's skin requires protection, blood pressure measurements obtained before and after the skin protectant is applied should be compared to determine differences.
	Initially, remove the cuff to inspect the skin after 1 hour of frequent use of the monitor. Thereafter, inspect the skin and extremity distal to the cuff every 4 hours.	Observing for possible venous pooling and congestion caused by use of an NIBP device is important. Indications are pain and skin discoloration and coolness. Excessive venous pressure can lead to tissue ischemia and nerve damage.			
	For continuous monitoring, the time between inflations should be set at 5 minutes or more.	Longer intervals between cuff inflations make venous congestion less likely.			
	For patients with delicate, fragile skin, a thin layer of gauze or stockinette can be used between the cuff and the skin.	A thin layer of protection between cuff and skin may decrease skin injury.			
Quality Control Issues	Calibration may be recommended to ensure accuracy.	NIBP monitor offsets (a compensating equivalent) can lead to erroneous BP measurement.	I: Manufacturer's recommendation only	Product manufacturer's operating manual	Refer to product manufacturer's operating manual for specific information on calibration.

Period of Use	Recommendation	Rationale for Recommendation	Level of Recommendation	Supporting References	Comments
Quality Control Issues (*cont.*)	Inspect cuffs for leaks and excessive grime or moisture before using them.	The cuff could serve as a medium for bacterial growth and possibly lead to infection of the patient.		See Other References: 1, 2, 3, 4	
	Inspect tubings for leaks and kinks before using them.	Leaks in the tubing or cuff can lead to malfunction of the monitor.			Many of the NIBP troubleshooting suggestions listed in the operator's manual instruct the user to check the cuff and tubing connections for leaks or kinks when the device fails to measure blood pressure.
	When machine malfunction is suspected, check the patient's condition first before troubleshooting the device.				
Potential Occupational Hazards	Follow manufacturer's directions for connecting the device to the patient and the monitor to the power source.	Correct connections ensure safe operation of the device.	I: Manufacturer's recommendation only		
	Inspect the power cord and plug for frays, breaks, and loose prongs before use.	Proper maintenance of the equipment prevents potential disruption in electrical connection and resultant monitor malfunction. It also prevents potential shocks, sparks, and electrical fires.			
	Assess the monitor's carrying handles and pole mount adapters for stability before transport.	Properly attached handles and adapters prevent injury to personnel and patients from a dropped or falling monitor.			

ANNOTATED BIBLIOGRAPHY

1. Derrico DJ. Comparison of blood pressure measurement methods in critically ill children. *Dimens Crit Care Nurs.* 1993;12(1):31–39.

Study Sample

Hemodynamically stable infants and children (n = 12); age range, 2 weeks to 16 years.

Comparison Studied

Direct arterial, oscillometric, and Doppler measurements of blood pressure.

Study Procedures

For each subject, investigators continuously monitored arterial blood pressure in 1 extremity and compared the direct measurements with 3 oscillometric measurements and 3 Doppler measurements of SBP in the other extremity.

Key Results

Thirty-six oscillometric and 36 Doppler measurements were compared with direct arterial measurements. Differences from direct arterial measurements were as follows: oscillometric systolic, 0–33 mm Hg; oscillometric mean, 1–36 mm Hg; oscillometric diastolic, 0–37 mm Hg; and Doppler systolic, 0–21 mm Hg. Doppler systolic readings corresponded to direct measurements of arterial systolic pressure more often than the oscillometric readings did. Of the oscillometric readings, the mean blood pressure was less likely to vary from the directly measured MAP. No significant differences were found between the Doppler or oscillometric measurements and the direct measurements.

Study Strengths and Weaknesses

Strengths: The subjects were infants and children. The investigators measured the circumference of the extremity to determine proper cuff size. Doppler and oscillometric methods are commonly used in pediatric units.

Weaknesses: The investigators did not determine if arm-to-arm differences in blood pressure existed in the subjects before the study. Movement of the extremity occurred during measurements of pressure. Indirect measurements of brachial blood pressure were compared with direct measurements of radial blood pressure and indirect measurements of calf blood pressure with direct measurements of dorsalis pedis blood pressure.

Clinical Implications

This study found clinically significant differences of up to 36 mm Hg between direct measurements of arterial blood pressure and indirect Doppler and oscillometric measurements of blood pressure in stable critically ill infants and children. The author indicates that the indirect measurements were higher than the direct measurements. He cites several variables that could have contributed to the higher indirect readings. For instance, indirect measurement of brachial blood pressure was compared with pressure in the radial artery; the latter is often higher in children because of peripheral amplification of blood pressure. As the artery narrows, the pressure increases, leading to higher blood pressures in the periphery. If peripheral amplification occurred in this study, the direct measurements of blood pressure in the radial artery would have been higher than the indirect measurements, so this is not a sound rationale for the higher indirect readings. The more likely cause of differences and overestimation with the oscillometric method was movement by the subjects. Movement of the subject during oscillometric determination of blood pressure can lead to erroneous measurements. The author notes that subjects moved during oscillometric determinations. These values should not have been included in the comparison with the direct arterial measures, because the oscillometric ones were likely not accurate when movement of the subject's arm occurred.

2. Venus B, Mathru M, Smith R, Pham, C. Direct versus indirect blood pressure measurements in critically ill patients. *Heart Lung.* 1985;14(3):228–231.

Study Sample

Hemodynamically unstable adults; mean age, 63 ± 12 years; 23 women and 20 men (n = 43).

Comparison Studied

Oscillometric NIBP measurements of blood pressure vs direct measurement of pressure in the radial artery (20-gauge arterial catheter).

Study Procedures

Arm-to-arm differences in blood pressure were ruled out. Direct measurements of blood pressure in the radial artery were compared with indirect measurements of blood pressure in the brachial artery obtained with the *appropriately* sized cuff. The SBP, DBP, and MAP were recorded simultaneously from the invasive and NIBP monitors for 3 consecutive 1-minute cycles of the NIBP monitor. Blood pressures were determined again when any hemodynamic change occurred.

Key Results

A total of 109 simultaneous measurements were taken. No significant differences were found between MAP determined directly or with the NIBP monitor. NIBP measurements of MAP (range, 53–163 mm Hg) were slightly higher than the direct measurements (range, 50–158 mm Hg). Significant differences were found for SBP and DBP. NIBP measurements of SBP (mean, 131 mm Hg) were lower than direct measurements (mean, 140 mm Hg). NIBP measurements of DBP (mean, 92 mm Hg) were higher than direct measurements (mean, 65 mm Hg).

Study Strengths and Weaknesses

Strengths: The investigation included measurements obtained during periods of hemodynamic instability, had a large sample size, and determined if arm-to-arm differences in blood pressure existed before subjects were studied.

Weaknesses: Subjects' diagnoses are not included in the sample description, and hemodynamic instability is not defined.

Clinical Implications

The authors do consider that the differences they found could be due to the fact that they were comparing radial blood pressure with brachial blood pressures. With the NIBP monitor used in this study, SBP was underestimated by an average of 9.2 mm Hg, and DBP was overestimated by an average of 8.7 mm Hg. These differences correspond to the physiologic differences between pressures in the brachial and radial arteries, but the authors do not think that the difference of 9 mm Hg is purely physiologic. Clinically, a difference of 9 mm Hg in SBP does not usually lead to changes in treatment, but a difference of 9 mm Hg in DBP could make a difference in treatment for hypertension. Additionally, the location where the blood pressure is being monitored (brachial, radial) must be taken into consideration when intervention is required.

3. Lehmann K, Gelman J, Weber M, Lafrades A. Comparative accuracy of three automated techniques in the noninvasive estimation of central blood pressure in men. *Am J Cardiol.* 1998;81(8):1004–1012.

Study Sample

Cardiovascular patients undergoing left heart catheterization for evaluation of chest pain syndromes (N = 120). All were male with an age range of 37–75 years.

Comparison Studied

Direct measurements of SBP, DBP, and MAP were done in the ascending aorta during cardiac catheterization using a leveled and calibrated, fluid-filled, commercially available system. For the noninvasive measurement, patients were randomized into 3 device groups, Device I (Dinamap 1846SX, Critikon Inc., Tampa, Fla), Device II (Accutorr 1a, Datascope Corp, Paramus, NJ) and Device III (Paramed 9200, Paramed Technology Inc, Mountain View, Calif).

Study Procedures

Invasive blood pressures in the ascending aorta were recorded continuously and marked during each of the comparison noninvasive blood pressure measurements. Five blood pressure measurements were obtained in each patient, with 2 minutes between each measurement, for a total of 600 measurements. All noninvasive devices were calibrated prior to data collection according to manufacturer recommendations. Data collectors were blinded to the central blood pressure measurement.

Key Results

Interrater reliability for the invasive blood pressure measurement ranged from 0.26 to 0.44, with a maximum difference of 3mm Hg. The automated devices were better at predicting diastolic pressure than they were for systolic or mean, with average absolute errors of 6.0, 7.4, and 6.8 mm Hg, respectively. Device I with oscillometric detection and stepped deflation was statistically more accurate than the other 2 devices, which used the automated ausculatory method. With all patients and devices combined, there was a slight trend toward overestimation of mean and diastolic pressure (p < .0001), but not systolic (p = NS). Clinically signification errors of greater than 20 mm Hg occurred 3.2% of the time, and were the least frequent with Device I than with either of the other 2 devices.

Study Strengths and Weaknesses

Strengths: Gold reference standard was used, and all invasive blood pressure tracings were checked for damping prior to be used as a comparison for the noninvasive measurements. A computer generated random number table was used for noninvasive device group assignment. Interrater reliability testing was done for the invasive reference blood pressure measurements.

Weaknesses: All subjects were male, limiting the generalization of the findings across gender. Because of the patient population used, 1/3 of the readings were done at blood pressures in excess of 140/90. In addition, no extreme values were used (i.e., cardiogenic shock patients or malignant hypertension). It was not specified whether the patients in the study were inpatients, outpatients, or a combination. Finally, only a 2 minute waiting period between NIBP measures was used, possibly contributing some error to the results.

Clinical Implications

This study evaluated 3 different noninvasive blood pressure monitors in a cardiac catherization laboratory setting. Because this study was done under ideal conditions in a controlled setting, it is possible that the findings do not accurately reflect what you might find during routine clinical use. Also, even though the results were statistically significant, the largest difference in absolute error was only 1.4 mm Hg, which is not clinically significant.

4. Mundt K, Chambless L, Burnham C, Heiss G. Measuring ankle systolic blood pressure: validation of the DINAMAPÔ 1846SX. *Angiology.* 1992;43(7):555–566.

Study Sample

Male and female volunteer subjects without vascular disease; age range, 23 to 67 years (N = 72).

Comparison Studied

Doppler and oscillometric NIBP measurements of SBP in the ankle of the same leg were compared. Techniques of wrapping the ankle cuff (contour vs parallel) were also compared for their effect on accuracy.

Study Procedures

Four measurements of SBP in the ankle were obtained for each type of cuff wrap at 60-second intervals. With the contour wrap, the edges of the cuff followed the contour of the ankle/leg. With the parallel wrap, the cuff edges ran perpendicular to the leg. For both types, the cuff was placed 2 in above the malleolus. A registered vascular technologist obtained Doppler measurements of SBP from the posterior tibial artery on the same leg at the same time that the oscillometric monitor was used to determine blood pressure in the ankle. The cuff used with the monitor had a pressure transducer attached so that the Doppler measurement of SBP could be determined simultaneously.

Key Results

Measurement of SBP was more precise with the contour wrap, and the oscillometric monitor gave accurate determinations of SBP. The oscillometric measurements of SBP in the ankle were less variable than those obtained with Doppler sonography, which is the standard method for determining blood pressure in the lower extremity. Doppler measurements of SBP varied more according to the type of cuff wrap than oscillometric measurements did. The values (mean, 3.0 mm Hg) obtained with the oscillometric monitor were lower that those obtained with the Doppler method.

Study Strengths and Weaknesses

Strengths: The study had a large number of subjects. Oscillometric and Doppler measurements of pressure were done on the same leg at the same time. The effect of the way the cuff was wrapped was considered.

Weaknesses: Subjects were healthy volunteers. The researchers did not obtain measurements of blood pressure in the upper extremity at the same time for comparisons.

Clinical Implications

Accurate measurements of SBP can be obtained from the ankle with the type of oscillometric monitor used in this study. This is useful information when determining if patients have differences in blood pressure in the ankle vs the arm (to determine peripheral vascular disease) or when measurement of blood pressure in the brachial artery is not possible. The manufacturer recommends that the ankle be used rather than the thigh because use of the ankle is more comfortable for the patient. If the patient is in shock or has peripheral vascular disease, the ankle should not be used to determine blood pressure, because further compromise to the extremity can occur.

5. Rutten AJ, Ilsley AH, Skowronski GA, Runcman WB. A comparative study of the measurement of mean arterial blood pressure using automatic oscillometers, arterial cannulation and auscultation. *Anaesth Intensive Care.* 1986;14(1):58–65.

Study Sample

Patients undergoing elective abdominal aortic surgery (n = 60).

Comparison Studied

Direct measurements of MAP in the radial artery were compared with measurements of MAP obtained with 6 automatic oscillometric devices. Additionally, in 15 subjects, measurements obtained with auscultation were compared with those obtained with 1 oscillometric device.

Study Procedures

Mean arterial pressure was measured directly in the radial artery (averaged over a period of 10 heart beats), then indirectly in the brachial artery (cuff width, 40% of arm circumference), and then directly again in the radial artery. The 2 direct measurements were averaged and compared with the indirect measurement. This procedure was repeated for all 6 devices on each subject. Nurses in the ICU used auscultation to determine SBP and DBP once before and once after automatic determination of blood pressure with a specified device. The values obtained with auscultation were averaged and compared with values obtained with the oscillometric devices.

Key Results

With all 6 devices, MAP tended to be overestimated, especially for lower MAP values. For all 6 devices, the average difference between direct and indirect measurements was less than 5 mm Hg (total of 1947 measurements). The authors note that a single indirect measurement could vary greatly (−29% to +40%) from the direct measurement. In addition, measurements of MAP in a patient in atrial fibrillation were difficult to compare because of the beat-to-beat variation. The SBP and DBP values obtained by auscultation by the ICU nurses were within 1 mm Hg of those obtained with the oscillometric monitor.

Study Strengths and Weaknesses

Strengths: The study compared measurements obtained with all 6 devices with direct measurement of MAP for each patient and used a large number of subjects and comparisons.

Weaknesses: Direct and indirect measurements of MAP were not obtained simultaneously. Measurements obtained by the oscillometric method were compared with measurements obtained with auscultation for only 1 device. Measurements of SBP and DBP were not compared.

Clinical Implications

The clinical usefulness of monitoring MAP trends is not recognized by all critical care units, because many units follow trends in SBP and DBP. A difference of 5 mm Hg in MAP is usually not critical unless the MAP falls below 65 mm Hg. Mean arterial pressure tended to be overestimated with all 6 noninvasive devices tested, especially when the MAP was low (50–75 mm Hg). Clinically, these findings indicate that NIBP devices should not be relied on for accurate determination of MAP when the MAP is low, a situation in which accuracy may be most crucial. The authors of this study do indicate that because of the beat-to-beat variations, determination of blood pressure with NIBP monitors that use the oscillometric technique may not be reliable when a patient has atrial fibrillation or an irregular heart beat. Another important consideration is that a single NIBP determination of MAP can vary greatly from the MAP determined by an invasive method. Treatment decisions should not be based on a single NIBP determination; complete assessment of the patient should be included.

6. Kaufmann MA, Pargger H, Drop LJ. Oscillometric blood pressure measurements by different devices are not interchangeable. *Anesth Analg.* 1996;82(2):377–381.

Study Sample

Inpatients with major depression were studied during ECT administration (N = 25).

Comparison Studied

Two Dinamap devices with identical software (model 1846SX, Critikon, Tampa, Fla) were compared. One device (SpL) was in a SpaceLabs Monitor (Redmond, Va) and the other (Marq) was in a Marquette Monitor (Marquette Electronics, Milwaukee, Wis).

Study Procedures

Two groups of patients were studied. In group 1, SpL (12 patients, 182 data points), blood pressure measurements were compared in 4 consecutive ECT treatments. In group 2, Marq (13 patients, 193 data points), blood pressure measurements were also compared in 4 consecutive ECT treatments. Bias and variability were tested for acceptable agreement between the 2 groups

Key Results

For the SpL group, SBP and MAP were within the AAMI criteria, diastolic was not. For the Marq group, all blood pressures were within AAMI criteria.

Study Strengths and Weaknesses

Strengths: Computerized data collection.

Weaknesses: Sample size was small, procedures were not at all well described. It is very difficult to figure out what the investigators in the study even compared, except by reading the results section. Convenience sampling used. The time intervals between the blood pressure readings were not specified. Standard cuff sizes were used on all patients, position of arm relative to supine patient position was not described.

Clinical Implications

Because both the study procedure and sample characteristics were poorly described, it is difficult to make any clinical recommendations from the findings. However, the question regarding clinical comparison between commercially available oscillometric NIBP devices is definitely worthy of further clinical investigation.

7. Park MK, Menard SM. Accuracy of blood pressure measurement by the DINAMAPÔ monitor in infants and children. *Pediatrics.* 1987;79(6):907–914.

Study Sample

Pediatric intensive care patients (n = 29); age range, 1 month to 16 years; the majority were studied after open heart surgery for repair of congenital heart defects.

Comparison Studied

Direct measurement of blood pressure in the radial artery vs indirect measurement with an oscillometric device. In 20 of the subjects, direct measurements were also compared with measurements obtained by an auscultatory method.

Study Procedures

In sedated patients, on the arm opposite the radial arterial line, blood pressure was measured once with the oscillometric device and then once by using the auscultatory method.

Key Results

The ranges of blood pressure in the radial artery were SBP, 81 to 131 mm Hg; DBP, 38 to 78 mm Hg; and MAP, 54 to 94 mm Hg. The differences between the indirect oscillometric measurements and the direct measurements were less for SBP (-7 to $+7$ mm Hg) than for DBP (-10 to $+8$ mm Hg) and MAP (-10 to $+8$ mm Hg). The differences between measurements obtained with the auscultatory method and direct measurements were -14 to $+19$ mm Hg for SBP and -2 to $+22$ mm Hg for DBP.

Study Strengths and Weaknesses

Strengths: The investigators studied a wide age range of infants and children and compared simultaneous measurements.

Weaknesses: The investigators did not determine if arm-to-arm differences in blood pressure existed, especially in patients with congenital heart defects. A single NIBP measurement was compared with direct measurements of arterial blood pressure, and brachial NIBP determinations were compared with direct determinations of pressure in the radial artery.

Clinical Implications

This study showed that in stable infants and children, of the 2 NIBP methods compared with direct measurement of arterial blood pressure, the values obtained with the oscillometric method more closely approximated those obtained by direct measurement than values obtained with the auscultatory method did. Clinically, blood pressure can be difficult to auscultate in infants and children, and only SBP can be determined by Doppler or palpation methods of NIBP. The oscillometric method provides a way in infants and children to determine DBP noninvasively that gives values that closely approximate those obtained by direct measurement of arterial blood pressure.

8. Bur A, Hirschl MM, Herkner H, Oschatz E, Kofler J, Woisetschlager C, Laggner AN. Accuracy of oscillometric blood pressure measurement according to the relation between cuff size and upper-arm circumference in critically ill patients. *Crit Care Med.* 2000;28(2):371–376.

Study Sample

Critically ill adult patients (N = 38) admitted to the Emergency Department and requiring invasive blood pressure monitoring. Subjects were both male (N = 23) and female (N = 15) with an age range of 16–88 years, mean 58 ± 17. All subjects were intubated and receiving mechanical ventilation. APACHE II scores ranged from 12 to 32, with a mean of 22 ± 5 points.

Comparison Studied

Direct measurement of MAP in the radial artery vs oscillometric measurement of MAP in the brachial artery using different cuff sizes.

Study Procedures

All patients were in a supine position with both arms kept at the level of the heart. Prior to data collection the mid-upper-arm circumference was measured. Patients were divided into 3 groups according to upper-arm measurements. Group 1: 18–25 cm (n = 5), Group 2: 25.1–33 cm (n = 23), and Group 3: 33.1–47.5 cm (n = 10). After a resting period of 15 minutes oscillometric blood pressure measurements were performed at least every 3 minutes until 10–20 measurements with each of 3 different cuffs (Hewlett-Packard Cuff 40401, B, C, and D) were obtained on each patient in the study. The corresponding invasive arterial blood pressures were obtained simultaneously.

Key Results

Overall, 1494 pairs of simultaneous oscillometric and invasive blood pressure measurements were collected in 3-minute intervals from the 38 patients over a total of 72.3 hours. Mean sample time was 118 ± 41 minutes (range 54–285) and the mean arterial blood pressure during the study period was 86 ± 16 mm Hg (range 35–165). Across all measures, there was a significant difference between blood pressure obtained by invasive reference and those obtained noninvasively (p < .0001). In each patient group, blood pressure underestimation increased as the cuff size increased. Of the 539 blood pressure measurements obtained with the appropriate size cuff, the mean difference was -6.7 mm Hg, which was statistically significant (p < .0001).

For measurements where smaller than recommended blood pressure cuffs were used (333 measurements), the overall difference was -3.6 mmHg and was significant as well (p < .0001). These same findings also occurred in patients receiving inotropic blood pressure support. In 39% (n = 587) of the measurements, the difference between invasive and noninvasive blood pressure was less than 10 mm Hg. In 26% (n = 395), the difference was between 10 and 19.9 mm Hg and in 39% (n = 512) the difference was greater than 20 mm Hg.

Study Strengths and Weaknesses

Strengths: The investigators were careful to take all invasive and noninvasive blood pressure measurements according to recommended standards, and described their methods well. Statistical analyses were also well-described. Investigators used a gold standard and mean arterial pressure for comparison.

Weaknesses: In order to understand the blood pressure cuff sizes used, the reader would have to be familiar with Hewlett-Packard blood pressure cuffs. The sizes should have been specified according to AHA criteria. The waiting period of only 3 minutes between noninvasive measurements may not have been enough time to minimize the venous congestion that can be caused by noninvasive blood pressure measurement. Group sizes were different, patient population was not uniform, and a convenience sampling method was used.

Clinical Implications

While it is not specifically stated, since patients with irregular heart rates and rhythms were not excluded they are likely included in the study sample. This may have contributed to the differences in the blood pressure measurements, since other research has shown oscillometric measurements to be less accurate in this patient group. It is also important to keep in mind that 82% were on vasoactive blood pressure support, although analyses showed no differences in the results between patients with and without inotropic support. It is possible that the differences between the invasive and noninvasive blood pressure measurements were due to the NIBP algorithm, cuff sizes, or measurement error. While the authors suggest that the AHA cuff size recommendations may need reconsideration, more broadly these results support that oscillometric blood pressure measure has limitations in critically ill patients.

9. Bur A. Herkner H, Vlcek M, Woisetschlager C, Derhaschnig U, Delle Karth, G, Laggner AN. Factors influencing the accuracy of oscillometric blood pressure measurement in critically ill patients. *Crit Care Med.* 2003;31(3):793-799.

Study Sample

Critically ill adult patients (N = 30) admitted to the Emergency Department and requiring invasive blood pressure monitoring. Subjects were both male (N = 17) and female (N = 13) with an age range of 21–82 years, mean 58 ± 12. APACHE II scores ranged from 14 to 31, with a mean of 21 ± 4 points. Sixty-seven percent of the patients were receiving inotropic blood pressure support and all patients were mechanically ventilated.

Comparison Studied

Direct measurement of MAP in the radial artery vs oscillometric measurement of MAP in the brachial artery using different cuff sizes and a new oscillometric algorithm. Patients with greater than a 5 mm Hg difference between their right and left arm by the auscultatory method were excluded from the study.

Study Procedures

All patients were in a supine position with both arms kept at the level of the heart. Prior to data collection the mid-upper-arm circumference was measured. Patients were divided into 3 groups according to upper-arm measurements. Group 1: 18–25 cm (N = 10), Group 2: 25.1–33 cm (N = 10), and Group 3: 33.1–47.5 cm (N = 10). After a resting period of 15 minutes oscillometric blood pressure measurements were performed every 5 minutes on the right and left arm until 10–20 measurements with each of 3 different cuffs (Hewlett-Packard Cuff 40401, B, C, and D) was obtained on each patient in the study. The corresponding invasive arterial blood pressures were obtained simultaneously.

Key Results

Overall, 1011 pairs of simultaneous oscillometric and invasive blood pressure measurements were collected in 5-minute intervals from the 30 patients over a total of 82.1 hours. Mean sample time was 164 ± 17 minutes (range 120–205) and the mean arterial blood pressure during the study period was 81 ± 13 mm Hg (range 49–133). Across all measures, there was a significant difference between blood pressure obtained by invasive reference and those obtained noninvasively by both the new and the old algorithm. In each patient group, blood pressure underestimation increased as the cuff size increased.

The overall bias of −2.4 mm Hg obtained by the new algorithm was significantly lower that the bias established for the old algorithm (−5.3 mm Hg), and fully meets the AAMI standards.

Study Strengths and Weaknesses

Strengths: The investigators were careful to take all invasive and noninvasive blood pressure measurements according to recommended standards, and described their methods well. Statistical analyses were also well-described. Investigators used a gold standard and mean arterial pressure for comparison. Groups were of equal size, and the recommended 5-minute waiting period between noninvasive blood pressure measurements was used.

Weaknesses: In order to understand the blood pressure cuff sizes used, the reader would have to be familiar with Hewlett-Packard blood pressure cuffs. The sizes should have been specified according to AHA criteria. The patient population was not uniform, and a convenience sampling method was used.

Clinical Implications

These data support that the new algorithm improves the accuracy of the oscillometric method. Data also continues to support the importance of appropriate cuff size during oscillometric blood pressure measurement. It is possible that the differences between the invasive and noninvasive blood pressure measurements were due to the NIBP algorithm, cuff sizes, or measurement error. While the authors suggest that the AHA cuff size recommendations may need reconsideration, more broadly these results support that oscillometric blood pressure measure has limitations in critically ill patients.

OTHER REFERENCES

1. Ramsey M. Blood monitoring: automated oscillometric devices. *J Clin Monitoring*. 1991;7:56–67.
2. Perloff D, Grim C, Flack J, et al. Human blood pressure determination by sphygmomanometry. *Circulation*. 1993; 88(5):2460–2470.
3. McGee BH, Bridges EJ. Monitoring arterial blood pressure: what you may not know. *Crit Care Nurse*. 2002; 2(2):60–79.
4. Bridges EJ, Middleton R. Direct vs oscillometric monitoring of blood pressure: stop comparing and pick one (a decision-making algorithm). *Crit Care Nurse*. 1997;17(3):58–72.
5. Gibbs CR, Murray S, Beevers DG. The clinical value of ambulatory blood pressure monitoring. *Heart*. 1998;79(2):115–117.
6. Artinian NT. Innovations in blood pressure monitoring: new, automated devices provide in-home or around-the-clock readings. *Am J Nurs*. 2004;104(8):52–60.
7. Pickering TG. Principles and techniques of blood pressure measurement. *Cardiol Clin*. 2002;20(2):207–223.
8. Jones DW, Appel LJ, Sheps SG, et al. Measuring blood pressure accurately: new and persistent challenges. *JAMA*. 2003;289(8):1027–1030.

Pulse Oximetry Monitoring

Mary Jo Grap RN, PhD, ACNP, FAAN

CHAPTER FIVE

Pulse Oximetry Monitoring

CASE STUDY

Mr Halle is a 64-year-old man who was admitted to the medical-surgical unit because of chest pain on inspiration and dyspnea on exertion. He has a long medical history that includes chronic obstructive pulmonary disease, myocardial infarction 10 years ago, and borderline hypertension. Analysis of a blood sample obtained in the emergency department showed that his arterial blood gases were fairly representative of his normal baseline values. Pulse oximetry was initiated to monitor his oxygenation. After 2 hours on the unit, he complained of increasing dyspnea, and his SpO_2 began to drop. His vital signs were: blood pressure, 158/95 mm Hg; heart rate, 142 beats per minute; respirations, 30 breaths/min; and body temperature, 38.0°C. Auscultation indicated crackles in the right lower lobe of the lung and expiratory wheezes. Subsequently, pneumonia was diagnosed, mechanical ventilation was started, and Mr Halle was moved to the ICU. His oxygen saturation was monitored continuously with pulse oximetry.

After stabilization in the ICU, he complained of back discomfort, and in an effort to help him to a position of comfort, the head of the bed was lowered. However, his SpO_2, which had been stable at 90%, decreased to less than 85%. The head of the bed was elevated, and subsequent changes of position and monitoring of his SpO_2 showed that his best position for optimal oxygenation was a head elevation of at least 45°. Pulse oximetry was used to wean him from oxygen therapy. He maintained his oxygenation throughout his stay and was discharged from the ICU 2 days later.

GENERAL DESCRIPTION

Pulse oximetry is a method for the continuous noninvasive measurement of arterial oxygen saturation (SpO_2). By far

the greatest part of oxygen transported by the blood is bound to hemoglobin, and the degree of binding (the saturation) is determined by the percentage of hemoglobin that is loaded with oxygen. SpO_2 indicates the amount of hemoglobin that is saturated with oxygen. However, it does not provide any information about the amount of hemoglobin present, the adequacy of ventilation, or cardiac output, all of which are important for optimal tissue oxygenation.

Pulse oximeters detect and calculate the absorption of light by functional hemoglobin to produce a measurement, SpO_2, which is an estimate of SaO_2. Functional hemoglobin is active in the transport of oxygen: oxygenated hemoglobin and deoxygenated hemoglobin (also called reduced hemoglobin). Absorption of light by oxygenated hemoglobin differs from the absorption by deoxygenated hemoglobin. The sensor of a pulse oximeter contains a photodetector and two light-emitting diodes (LED), which emit two wavelengths of monochromatic light: red and infrared (Figure 5.1). The

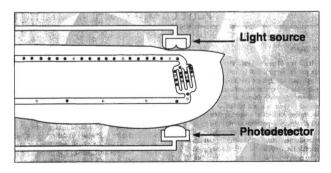

Figure 5.1 Placement of the photodetector and light-emitting diodes of a pulse oximetry sensor. Used with permission. Nellcor Puritan Bennett, Pleasanton, Calif.

two diodes alternate and cycle on and off many times per second. With this arrangement, a single detector can be used to sample first one wavelength and then the other. The absorption of light by hemoglobin is analyzed over a full pulse beat to make the saturation measurement independent of these factors. The total absorption of light has two components, a constant that accounts for tissue and steadily flowing venous blood and one that changes with arterial pulsation. In conventional oximetry, the value of the constant component is subtracted from the total value, so that the net absorption of each wavelength can be attributed to arterial blood only. Some "new generation" motion-tolerant pulse oximeters identify and isolate signals from venous blood as well as reduce motion artifact. The pulse oximeter analyzes the relative absorption of each waveform of light and provides a SpO_2 measurement. The saturation values that are displayed are averaged over several seconds.

ACCURACY

In numerous early studies, primarily on healthy volunteers, the accuracy of pulse oximetry over the range of 70% to 100% oxygen saturation has been substantiated. In general, when compared with arterial oxygen saturation (SaO_2), the accuracy of SpO_2 in clinical practice is good and is within ±2% for SaO_2 greater than 70%. In an analysis of pulse oximetry studies, the bias and precision for a total of 1447 paired measurements over a SaO_2 range of 51% to 100% were calculated. The accuracy was found to be clinically acceptable, defined as a bias of ±2% or less (range, −1.4% to +1.9%) and a precision of ±3% or less (range, ±1.6% to ±3.1%). Although earlier studies have shown decreased accuracy of SpO_2 in hypoxemia and hemodynamic instability, more recently, "new generation" pulse oximeters have improved signal detection algorithms and enhanced accuracy for oxygen saturations less than 70%, although data is limited. Motion artifact from patient movement can result in inaccurate values or false alarms. However, "new generation," motion tolerant pulse oximeters contain improved software that result in reduce false alarm frequency and improved accuracy when compared to conventional (older) pulse oximeters.

COMPETENCY

A clear understanding of oxygenation and ventilation is essential in caring for patients who are being monitored with pulse oximetry. Assuming that the patient's pulmonary status is stable as long as the pulse oximeter value is within normal limits can result in life-threatening conditions of hypoventilation and acid-base disturbances. Clinicians must understand the relationship between PaO_2 and SaO_2 as represented by the oxyhemoglobin dissociation curve. Several studies have described clinicians' lack of understanding of the principles of pulse oximetry monitoring, how it works,

and factors that affected the reading. It is important to understand that the relationship between PaO_2 and SaO_2 is not linear and that SaO_2 or SpO_2 may be relatively normal while PaO_2 drops significantly, emphasizing that SpO_2 is not a sensitive measure of oxygenation. In addition, this relationship is affected by changes in acid-base balance and temperature. Although SpO_2 is accurate and extremely useful in the clinical setting, it is but one part of the total assessment of a patient and should never be used as the sole monitor of the patient's oxygenation and ventilation status.

ETHICAL CONSIDERATIONS

Ethical considerations associated with the use of pulse oximetry are similar to those associated with any monitoring devices. It is the nurse's responsibility to understand indications for pulse oximetry, the factors that may affect accuracy and to act as the patient's advocate to ensure its appropriate use. In addition, nurses must be well trained in the care and application of the device and ensure that patients are protected from any adverse complications related to its use. To provide competent care, nurses must also have a complete understanding of the concepts underlying pulse oximetry and the resulting measurements.

OCCUPATIONAL HAZARDS

No specific occupational hazards are associated with the use of pulse oximeters. Potential hazards are similar to those associated with any electrical device.

FUTURE RESEARCH

Comprehensive evaluation of new generation pulse oximeters including reflectance technology using a forehead sensor is needed in a wide range of populations and in a variety of applications. Evaluation of educational programs to enhance pulse oximetry knowledge and its appropriate use should also be conducted. Most importantly, research is needed to describe specific patient outcomes that have been improved by the use of pulse oximetry or how care has been positively affected. These data are required to identify the appropriate use of this technology.

SUGGESTED READINGS

Ahrens T, Tucker K. Pulse oximetry. *Crit. Care Nurs Clin. North Am.* 1999;11:87–98.

Attin M, Cardin S, Dee V, Doering L, Dunn D, Ellstrom K, et al. An educational project to improve knowledge related to pulse oximetry. *Am J Crit Care.* 2002;11:529–534.

Keogh BF. When pulse oximetry monitoring of the critically ill is not enough. *Anesth Analg.* 2002;94:S96–S99.

Pedersen T, Pedersen P, Moller AM. Pulse oximetry for perioperative monitoring. The Cochrane Library. Oxford: Update Software; 2002.

Rotello LC, Warren J, Jastremski MS, Milewski A. A nurse-directed protocol using pulse oximetry to wean mechanically ventilated patients from toxic oxygen concentrations. *Am J Respir Crit Care Med.* 1992;102:1833–1835.

Seguin P, Le Rouzo A, Tanguy M, Guillou YM, Feuillu A, Malledant Y. Evidence for the need of bedside accuracy of pulse oximetry in an intensive care unit. *Crit Care Med.* 2000;28:703–706.

St. John RE, Thomson PD. Noninvasive respiratory monitoring. *Crit Care Nurs Clin North Am.* 1999;11: 423–435.

CLINICAL RECOMMENDATIONS

The rating scales for the Level of Recommendation column range from I to VI, with levels indicated as follows: I, manufacturer's recommendation only; II, theory based, no research data to support recommendations, recommendations from expert consensus group may exist; III, laboratory data only, no clinical data to support recommendations; IV, limited clinical studies to support recommendations; V, clinical studies in more than 1 or 2 different populations and situations to support recommendations; VI, clinical studies in a variety of patient populations and situations to support recommendations.

Period of Use	Recommendation	Rationale for Recommendation	Level of Recommendation	Supporting References	Comments
Selection of Patients	Pulse oximetry is recommended in the following circumstances.				
	In patients at risk for hypoxemia: those in inpatient and outpatient settings; during and after anesthesia, critically ill patients, especially patients who have marginal or fluctuating oxygenation or high FiO_2 or are receiving inotropes, vasopressors, vasodilators, sedatives, or analgesics. Its use is also recommended for monitoring of patients in the emergency department, both adults and children, who are at risk for oxygenation problems.	Desaturation is detected sooner by pulse oximetry than by clinical observation. Pulse oximetry is the standard of practice during and after anesthesia; its use increases detection of hypoxemia due to the effects of anesthetics, sedatives, relaxants, and opioids. Vasoactive medications can cause changes in oxygenation that may be detected more readily by pulse oximetry than by physical assessments. Pulse oximetry allows rapid detection of declining SaO_2 long before it is clinically apparent and may help in making triage decisions.	VI: Clinical studies in a variety of populations and situations	See Other References: 18–25	The American Association of Post Anesthesia Nurses recommends ongoing assessment of SpO_2 during the recovery period after anesthesia.
	Use pulse oximetry during invasive procedures: placement of central lines, bronchoscopy, endoscopy, and cardiac catheterization.	Risk of hypoxemia may be increased with use of the Trendelenburg position, use of drapes over the face that may compromise ventilation, longer procedures, and use of sedatives and analgesics during the procedure.	V: Clinical studies in more than 1 or 2 different populations and situations to support recommendations	See Other References: 2, 26–28	
	Use pulse oximetry during weaning from mechanical ventilation, use of continuous positive airway pressure, and to evaluate oxygen use and titration.	Pulse oximetry may be used in place of analysis of arterial blood gases during weaning from mechanical ventilation and oxygen titration.	VI: Clinical studies in a variety of populations and situations	See Other References: 2, 12, 29–34	If discrepancies between pulse oximetry and the patient's clinical picture occur, arterial blood gases should be obtained to verify pulse oximetry values.

Period of Use	Recommendation	Rationale for Recommendation	Level of Recommendation	Supporting References	Comments
Selection of Patients (*cont.*)	Use pulse oximetry in adults and children during transport from the operating room to postanesthesia recovery, during travel outside the ICU and during ambulance travel to evaluated need for oxygen therapy.	Significant hypoxemia can occur during transport. Use of pulse oximetry during ambulance travel has reduced cost by decreasing oxygen use.	VI: Clinical studies in a variety of populations and situations	See Other References: 35–38	Guidelines (American Association of Critical Care Nurses and Society of Critical Care Medicine) for transport of critically ill patients include continuous pulse oximetry monitoring with periodic documentation of SpO_2.
	Pulse oximetry may be less useful for monitoring hyperoxemia in neonates, for use in patients with low arterial oxygen saturation (less than 70%), in the presence of dyshemoglobins such as methemoglobin and carboxy hemoglobin, and in patients with severe anemia.	Pulse oximetry may be inadequate for monitoring hyperoxemia in premature neonates. Due to the shape of the oxygen dissociation curve where large changes in PaO_2 are associated with very small changes in SaO_2, pulse oximetry has limited sensitivity in the highest saturation ranges. In patients with arterial oxygen saturation less than 70%, pulse oximetry may be more valuable as a tool for showing trends since reliability may be affected. In the presence of dyshemoglobins such as methemaglobin and carboxyhemoglobin, SpO_2 measures are less reliable measures of SaO_2. Measurements must be interpreted in light of the patient's clinical features. When clinically significant levels of dyshemoglobins are present, analysis of arterial blood gases should regularly accompany assessments. Pulse oximeters may not provide SpO_2 measurements when the level of hemoglobin is less than 3 to 5 g/dL.	VI: Clinical studies in a variety of populations and situations	See Other References: 25, 30, 39–47	New generation pulse oximeters may be better able to detect hyperoxemia, a danger in neonates that results in retinopathy and chronic lung disease. The pulsatile fraction of total light from the ears is smaller than that from the fingers (the site used most often). In patients with peripheral vasoconstriction or hypotension, the ear or forehead (reflectance technology) may be used, although data concerning accuracy is conflicting. The ear lobe is the least vasoactive site and therefore the least susceptible to signal loss due to vasoconstriction. Levels of carboxyhemoglobin are increased in smokers due to inhalation of carbon monoxide. Levels of methemoglobin can be increased by use of nitrates, chlorates, antimalarials, sodium nitroprusside, and lidocaine. Although some authors have found that sufficient hemoglobin must be present in the blood for accurate oximeter function, others have found pulse oximetry to be accurate at low hemoglobin levels.
Application of Device and Initial Use	Choose the site with the best pulsatile vascular bed. (Figures 5.2–5.8)	In usual situations, the overall performance of finger sensors is generally better than the performance of sensors in other sites. Blood flow to a cannulated extremity may be compromised compared to a non-cannulated site negatively affecting the pulsatile	V: Clinical studies in more than 1 or 2 different populations and situations to support recommendations	See Other References: 48–52	Sensors are not interchangeable among all sites. Following manufacturer's recommendation for use and site placement will enhance accuracy. Because pulse oximeters cannot report data unless a pulse is

(continued)

(continued)

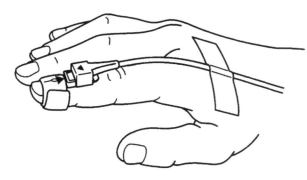

Figure 5.2   Finger placement of a pulse oximetry sensor. Used with permission. Nellcor Puritan Bennett, Pleasanton, Calif.

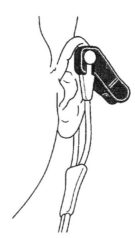

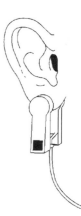

Figure 5.3   Sensor placement on the pinna of the ear. Used with permission. Nellcor Puritan Bennett, Pleasanton, Calif.

Figure 5.4   Sensor placement on the ear lobe. Used with permission. Nellcor Puritan Bennett, Pleasanton, Calif.

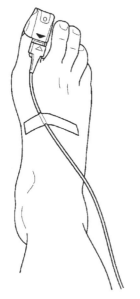

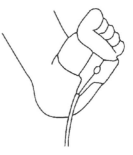

Figure 5.6   Sensor placement on the foot of an infant. Used with permission. Nellcor Puritan Bennett, Pleasanton, Calif.

Figure 5.5   Sensor placement on the toe. Used with permission. Nellcor Puritan Bennett, Pleasanton, Calif.

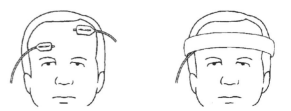

Figure 5.7   Sensor placement on the forehead. Used with permission. Nellcor Puritan Bennett, Pleasanton, Calif.

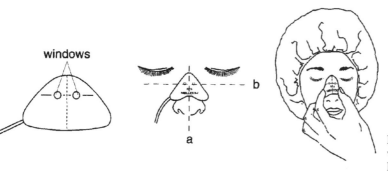

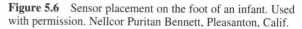

Figure 5.8   Sensor placement on the nose. Used with permission. Nellcor Puritan Bennett, Pleasanton, Calif.

Period of Use	Recommendation	Rationale for Recommendation	Level of Recommendation	Supporting References	Comments
Application of Device and Initial Use (*cont.*)		signal. During vasoconstriction of hypotension, use of adhesive sensors may improve signal quality or use of nose sensors may provide a faster response. However, correct placement using the nose sensor is critical for alignment of optical components. Manufacturers generally recommend use of the foot for infants.			flow to the sensor site by warming the extremity may enhance the pulse signal and facilitate detection of a pulse. This will not inflate SpO_2 values.
	When using the finger or toes as the monitoring site, remove nail polish (especially blue, black, green, or brown/red) and synthetic nails, particularly when pulsatile flow is not detected.	Certain colors and synthetic nails can cause errors of 3% to 6% in SpO_2 readings.	V: Clinical studies in more than 1 or 2 different populations and situations to support recommendations	See Other References: 53–58	There is conflicting evidence of the effect of nail polish and synthetic nails on pulse oximetry accuracy, but it is probably prudent to remove dark-colored polish whenever possible.
	The accuracy of oximetric readings can be transiently diminished in the presence of intravenous dyes.	Injected methylene blue and indocyanine green can produce transient false desaturation.	V: Clinical studies in more than 1 or 2 different populations and situations to support recommendations	See Other References: 56, 57, 59, 60	
	Extraneous light (e.g., infrared heat lamps, fluorescent light phototherapy) may affect accuracy. Reduce this effect by covering the sensor with opaque material.	Light that is very strong or flickering may, at frequencies similar to those of the LED, interfere with SpO_2 measurements.	V: Clinical studies in more than 1 or 2 different populations and situations to support recommendations	See Other References: 61–65	Although this is a theoretical concern, early studies were largely based on anecdotal reports. A recent evaluation found no significant effect on pulse oximetry readings.
Ongoing Monitoring	Optimal SpO_2 is 95% or greater, SpO_2 less than 90% reflects desaturation. SpO_2 should be interpreted in light of the patient's clinical features.	With normal dissociation of oxygen, SpO_2 of 95% or greater reflects a PaO_2 of 70 mm Hg or greater, and SpO_2 of less than 90% reflects a PaO_2 of 60 mm Hg or less.	V: Clinical studies in more than 1 or 2 different populations and situations to support recommendations	See Other References: 3, 30, 33, 66–68	During acid-base imbalances and alterations in temperature and PCO_2, the normal relationship between SaO_2 and PaO_2 is altered. Optimal SaO_2 levels in the neonate to both provide adequate oxygenation and reduce the risks of hyperoxemia have yet to be determined.
	Base nursing care decisions on SpO_2 trends and clinical assessment rather than on isolated values.	Individual, isolated values are not as representative of a patient's arterial oxygenation status as those provided by close monitoring of SpO_2 over time. Changes in body position and sensor movement can result in isolated changes in SpO_2. A consistent and sustained decrease in SpO_2 is more likely to indicate changes in a patient's status. When SpO_2 values and the clinical picture are inconsistent, evaluate oxygenation with arterial blood gas sampling.	V: Clinical studies in more than 1 or 2 different populations and situations to support recommendations	See Other References: 25, 69–71	

Period of Use	Recommendation	Rationale for Recommendation	Level of Recommendation	Supporting References	Comments
Prevention of Complications	Inspect or move the site of spring-tension sensors and adhesive sensors according to manufacturer's recommendations, generally every 8 hours for adhesive sensor sites and every 4 hours for reusable sensor sites.	Pulse oximeter induced digital injury including skin breakdown, burns, and ischemic necrosis at sensor placement sites occur approximately 5% of the time.	IV: Limited clinical studies to support recommendations	See Other References: 72–76	
Quality Control Issues	Routinely assess staff understanding of pulse oximetry concepts.	Deficiencies in knowledge and understanding of pulse oximetry persist in both nursing and medical staff.	V: Clinical studies in more than 1 or 2 different populations and situations to support recommendations	See Other References: 16, 77, 78	
	Clearly document pulse oximetry values as SpO_2 to distinguish SpO_2 values from SaO_2 measurements derived from analysis of arterial blood gases.	Although measurements of SaO_2 and SpO_2 are highly correlated, they are obtained in different ways (analysis of arterial blood gases and pulse oximetry), and in some circumstances, the values may be different. It is therefore prudent to differentiate between the two types of measurements.	II: Theory based, no research data to support recommendations; recommendations from expert consensus group may exist;	See Other References: 1, 57, 70	
	Continually assess the need for pulse oximetry.	Although identification of hypoxemia is increased with pulse oximetry use, there are few data that show improved patient outcomes (post-operative complications, length of stay, or mortality) using this technology.	VI: Clinical studies in a variety of patient populations and situations to support recommendations	See Other References: 12, 22–24, 79	The use of pulse oximetry is ubiquitous; however, the requirement for continuous monitoring should be evaluated frequently in every patient.
	Include pulse oximetry measurement as only one part of a total assessment of oxygenation and ventilation.	SpO_2 indicates the amount of hemoglobin that is saturated with oxygen. It does not provide any information about the amount of hemoglobin present, the adequacy of ventilation, or cardiac output. To best assess tissue oxygenation, all these factors must be evaluated.	IV: Limited clinical studies to support recommendations	See Other References: 80–82	

ANNOTATED BIBLIOGRAPHY

Literally hundreds of studies present various aspects of use of pulse oximetry. This bibliography provides an example from each area that is presently under study or has the greatest clinical impact, including pulse oximetry knowledge level, use during weaning, new technology, and effect on outcomes.

1. Attin M, Cardin S, Dee V, Doering L, Dunn D, Ellstrom K, et al. An educational project to improve knowledge related to pulse oximetry. *Am J Crit Care:* 2002;11:529–534.

Study Sample

442 staff members, 331 nurses, 82 physicians, and 29 respiratory therapists.

Comparison Studied

A test/survey of 17 true-false questions based on the research-based practice protocol of the American Association of Critical-Care Nurses was developed to evaluate current knowledge of pulse oximetry.

Study Procedures

This sample of medical, nursing, and respiratory therapy staff was invited to complete the test/survey before and several months after an educational program to improve staff members' knowledge of pulse oximetry. The program included educational forums, policy changes, competency checklists, and verification of inclusion of research-based principles in orientation programs.

Key Results

The overall percent of correct answers was 66%. Differences between disciplines were significant: respiratory therapists scored slightly higher (76%) than did nurses (64%) and physicians (66%) (P = .01). The scores on the test/survey given after the educational program increased significantly, from 66% to 82% (P < .01).

Study Strengths and Weaknesses

This study evaluated knowledge based on a protocol from a national authority (i.e. AACN) providing a good foundation for knowledge expectations and included several members of the multidisciplinary team. Although a local, convenience sample was used, which may include a majority of subjects who were motivated to learn, the sample size was large enough to increase validity of the data.

Clinical Implications

This study showed significant improvement in knowledge using a variety of methods that can easily be adapted to any setting.

2. Durbin CG, Jr., Rostow SK. More reliable oximetry reduces the frequency of arterial blood gas analyses and hastens oxygen weaning after cardiac surgery: a prospective, randomized trial of the clinical impact of a new technology. *Crit Care Med.* 2002;30:1735–1740.

Study Sample

The study enrolled 86 patients after undergoing coronary artery bypass surgery in a postcardiac surgery intensive care unit in a major teaching hospital.

Comparison Studied

The study evaluated the impact on clinical care of improved, innovative ("new generation") oximetry technology.

Study Procedures

All patients were monitored with two oximeters, one employing conventional oximetry (conventional pulse oximeter) and one using an improved innovative technology (innovative pulse oximeter), on different fingers of the same hand. The outputs from both devices were collected continuously by computer, but only one device was randomly selected and displayed for clinicians. The amount and percentage of nonfunctional monitoring time was collected.

Key Results

Amount and percentage of nonfunctional monitoring time was found to be much greater for the conventional pulse oximeter than the improved innovative technology; however, time to extubation was not different between the two oximeters. Clinicians managing patients with the more reliable improved innovative technology weaned patients faster to an FIO_2 of 0.40 and obtained fewer arterial blood gas measurements. But there were no differences in the number of ventilator changes during the weaning process between the oximeter.

Study Strengths and Weaknesses

This strong study design using the latest technology and focusing on care outcomes makes this a significant study.

Clinical Implications

Investigating the effect of a monitor on the process of care, rather than simply its accuracy and precision, is a useful, relevant approach for evaluating the impact of new technology.

3. Hummler HD, Engelmann A, Pohlandt F, Hogel J, Franz AR. Accuracy of pulse oximetry readings in an animal model of low perfusion caused by emerging pneumonia and sepsis. *Intensive Care Med.* 2004;30:709–713.

Study Sample

Twenty-five adult, anesthetized, ventilated rabbits.

Comparison Studied

To test the effects of low perfusion caused by emerging sepsis on the performance of two new pulse oximetry techniques: Masimo SET in comparison with Nellcor Oxismart XL using random allocation of two pulse oximetry devices to two sensor sites.

Study Procedures

Oxygen saturation was measured by pulse oximetry (SpO_2) and recorded continuously until death. Arterial oxygen saturation (SaO_2) was measured hourly by CO oximetry and whenever a difference of >5% between the devices occurred. SpO_2 sensors were positioned at both forelegs and switched hourly.

Key Results

There was no difference in total signal dropout time in Masimo SET vs Oxismart XL. There were fewer episodes with a false SpO_2 reading using the Masimo SET vs the Oxismart XL as verified by CO oximetry; $p < 0.05$. The difference between the SpO_2 and the SaO_2 was significant between the two devices.

Study Strengths and Weaknesses

Although this study used an animal model and provides data that may not be completely transferable to the human population, evaluation of pulse oximetry accuracy in low perfusion states is difficult in humans. Nonetheless this study provides excellent comparative data for the pulse oximeters used.

Clinical Implications

Both devices were able to pick up a signal and measure SpO_2 during most of the low perfusion time.

4. Moller JT, Johannessen NW, Espersen K, Ravlo O, Pedersen BD, Jensen PF, et al. Randomized evaluation of pulse oximetry in 20,802 patients: II. Perioperative events and postoperative complications. *Anesth.* 1993;78:445–453.

Study Sample

This study involved 20,802 surgical patients in Denmark who were randomly assigned to be monitored, or not, with pulse oximetry in the operating room (OR) and postanesthesia care unit (PACU).

Comparison Studied

The purpose of the study was to describe the effect of pulse oximetry monitoring on the frequency of unanticipated perioperative events, changes in patient care, and the rate of postoperative complications.

Study Procedures

Once assigned to receive pulse oximetry technology, or not, all types of critical events were documented both in the operating room and in the PACU. Anesthesiologists were also surveyed about their experience.

Key Results

There was a 19-fold increase in the incidence of diagnosed hypoxemia in the oximetry group over the control group in both the OR and PACU. Changes in PACU care with pulse oximetry use included higher flow rate of supplemental oxygen, increased use of supplemental oxygen at discharge, and increased use of naloxone. However, no significant differences in postoperative complications, duration of hospital stay, or number of hospital deaths were found between the two groups. Eighteen percent of anesthesiologists had experienced a situation in which a pulse oximeter helped to avoid a serious event or complication, and 80% felt more secure when they used a pulse oximeter.

Study Strengths and Weaknesses

This study is significant based on the prospective nature of data collection as well as the very large sample size. In addition, the comparison of events with and without pulse oximetry is also important, as this study would be almost impossible to conduct in the US due to ethical limitations based on a variety of practice guidelines that recommend pulse oximetry use.

Clinical Implications

Although this study showed that pulse oximetry can improve detection of hypoxemia in the OR and PACU and its use prompted changes in patient care, a reduction in the overall rate of postoperative complications was not observed. Pulse oximetry use should be continually assessed for its appropriate use.

OTHER REFERENCES

1. Severinghaus JW, Honda Y. History of blood gas analysis. VII. Pulse oximetry. *J Clin Monit.* 1987; 3:135–138.
2. Bierman MI, Stein KL, Snyder JV. Pulse oximetry in the postoperative care of cardiac surgical patients: a randomized controlled trail. *Am J Respir Crit Care Med.* 1992;102:1367–1370.
3. Seguin P, Le Rouzo A, Tanguy M, Guillou YM, Feuillu A, Malledant Y. Evidence for the need of bedside accuracy of pulse oximetry in an intensive care unit. *Crit Care Med.* 2000;28:703–706.
4. Technology Subcommittee of the Working Group on Critical Care. Noninvasive blood gas monitoring: a review for use in the adult critical care unit. *Can Med Assoc J.* 1992;146:703–721.

5. Benson JP, Venkatesh B, Patla V. Misleading information from pulse oximetry and the usefulness of continuous blood gas monitoring in a post cardiac surgery patient. *Intensive Care Med*. 1995;21:437–439.

6. Ibanez J, Velasco J, Raurich JM. The accuracy of the Biox 3700 pulse oximeter in patients receiving vasoactive therapy. *Intensive Care Med*. 1991;17:484–486.

7. Vicenzi MN, Gombotz H, Krenn H, Dorn C, Rehak P. Transesophageal versus surface pulse oximetry in intensive care unit patients. *Crit Care Med*. 2000; 28:2268–2270.

8. Hummler HD, Engelmann A, Pohlandt F, Hogel J, Franz AR. Accuracy of pulse oximetry readings in an animal model of low perfusion caused by emerging pneumonia and sepsis. *Intensive Care Med*. 2004; 30:709–713.

9. Irita K, Kai Y, Akiyoshi K, Tanaka Y, Takahashi S. Performance evaluation of a new pulse oximeter during mild hypothermic cardiopulmonary bypass. *Anesth Analg*. 2003;96:11–4, table.

10. Yamaya Y, Bogaard HJ, Wagner PD, Niizeki K, Hopkins SR. Validity of pulse oximetry during maximal exercise in normoxia, hypoxia, and hyperoxia. *J Appl Physiol*. 2002;92:162–168.

11. Durbin CG Jr, Rostow SK. Advantages of new technology pulse oximetry with adults in extremis. *Anesth Analg*. 2002;94:S81–S83.

12. Durbin CG Jr, Rostow SK. More reliable oximetry reduces the frequency of arterial blood gas analyses and hastens oxygen weaning after cardiac surgery: a prospective, randomized trial of the clinical impact of a new technology. *Crit Care Med*. 2002;30:1735–1740.

13. Lutter NO, Urankar S, Kroeber S. False alarm rates of three third-generation pulse oximeters in PACU, ICU and IABP patients. *Anesth Analg*. 2002;94:S69–S75.

14. Malviya S, Reynolds PI, Voepel-Lewis T, Siewert M, Watson D, Tait AR, Tremper K. False alarms and sensitivity of conventional pulse oximetry versus the Masimo SET technology in the pediatric postanesthesia care unit. *Anesth Analg*. 2000;90:1336–1340.

15. Davies G, Gibson AM, Swanney M, Murray D, Beckert L. Understanding of pulse oximetry among hospital staff. *N Z Med J*. 2003;116:U297.

16. Howell M. Pulse oximetry: an audit of nursing and medical staff understanding. *Br J Nurs*. 2002;11:191–197.

17. Stoneham MD, Saville GM, Wilson IH. Knowledge about pulse oximetry among medical and nursing staff. *Lancet*. 1994;344:1339–1342.

18. Cote C J. Pulse oximetry during conscious sedation. *JAMA*. 1994;271:429–430.

19. Eichhorn JH. Pulse oximetry as a standard of practice in anesthesia. *Anesth*. 1993;78:423–426.

20. Hanna D. Guidelines for pulse oximetry use in pediatrics. *J Pediatr Nurs*. 1995;10:124–126.

21. McKay WP, Noble WH. Critical incidents detected by pulse oximetry during anaesthesia. *Can J Anaesth*. 1988;35:265–269.

22. Moller JT. Anesthesia related hypoxemia. The effect of pulse oximetry monitoring on perioperative events and postoperative complications. *Dan Med Bull*. 1994; 41:489–500.

23. Moller JT, Johannessen NW, Espersen K, et al. Randomized evaluation of pulse oximetry in 20,802 patients: II. Perioperative events and postoperative complications. *Anesthesiology*. 1993;78:445–453.

24. Moller JT, Pedersen T, Rasmussen LS, et al. Randomized evaluation of pulse oximetry in 20, 802 patients: I. Design, demography, pulse oximetry failure rate, and overall complication rate. *Anesthesiology*. 1993;78: 436–444.

25. Severinghaus JW, Kelleher JF. Recent developments in pulse oximetry. *Anesthesiology*. 1992;76:1018–1038.

26. al-Hadeedi S, Leaper DJ. Falls in hemoglobin saturation during ERCP and upper gastrointestinal endoscopy. *World J Surg*. 1991;15:88–94.

27. Bendig DW. Pulse oximetry and upper intestinal endoscopy in infants and children. *J Pediatr Gastroenterol Nutr*. 1991;12:39–43.

28. Cote CJ, Rolf N, Liu LM, et al. A single-blind study of combined pulse oximetry and capnography in children. *Anesth*. 1991;74:980–987.

29. Inman KJ, Sibbald WJ, Rutledge FS, Speechley M, Martin CM, Clark BJ. Does implementing pulse oximetry in a critical care unit result in substantial arterial blood gas savings? *Am J Respir Crit Care Med*. 1993; 104:542–546.

30. Jubran A, Tobin MJ. Reliability of pulse oximetry in titrating supplemental oxygen therapy in ventilator-dependent patients. *Am J Respir Crit Care Med*. 1990; 97:1420–1425.

31. Marx WH, DeMaintenon NL, Mooney KF, et al. Cost reduction and outcome improvement in the intensive care unit. *J Trauma*. 1999;46:625–629.

32. Niehoff J, DelGuercio C, LaMorte W, et al. Efficacy of pulse oximetry and capnometry in postoperative ventilatory weaning. *Crit Care Med*. 1988;16:701–705.

33. Rotello LC, Warren J, Jastremski MS, Milewski A. A nurse-directed protocol using pulse oximetry to wean mechanically ventilated patients from toxic oxygen concentrations. *Am J Respir Crit Care Med*. 1992; 102:1833–1835.

34. Withington DE, Ramsay JG, Saoud AT, Bilodeau J. Weaning from ventilation after cardiopulmonary bypass: evaluation of a non-invasive technique. *Can J Anaesth*. 1991;38:15–19.

35. Guidelines for the transfer of critically ill patients. Guidelines Committee, American College of Critical Care Medicine, Society of Critical Care Medicine and the Transfer Guidelines Task Force. *Am J Crit Care*. 1993;2:189–195.

36. Elling A. *Oxygenation during preoperative transportation.* In Payne JP, Severinghaus JW, eds. Pulse Oximetry. Springer-Verlag, New York; 1995:161–164.

37. Howes DW, Field B, Leary T, Jones GR, Brison RJ. Justification of pulse oximeter costs for paramedic prehospital providers. *Prehosp Emerg Care.* 2000; 4:151–155.

38. Runcie CJ, Reeve W. Pulse oximetry during transport of the critically ill. *J Clin Monit.* 1991;7:348–349.

39. Awad AA, Ghobashy MA, Ouda W, Stout RG, Silverman DG, and Shelley KH. Different responses of ear and finger pulse oximeter wave form to cold pressor test. *Anesth Analg.* 2001;92:1483–1486.

40. Jay GD, Hughes L, Renzi FP. Pulse oximetry is accurate in acute anemia from hemorrhage. *Ann Emerg Med.* 1994;24:32–35.

41. Lee S, Tremper KK, Barker SJ. Effects of anemia on pulse oximetry and continuous mixed venous hemoglobin saturation monitoring in dogs. *Anesthesiology.* 1991;75:118–122.

42. Mannheimer PD, Bebout DE. The OxiMax System. Nellcor's new platform for pulse oximetry. *Minerva Anestesiol.* 2002;68:236–239.

43. Moyle JT. Uses and abuses of pulse oximetry. *Arch Dis Child.* 1996;74:77–80.

44. Poets CF, Urschitz MS, Bohnhorst B. Pulse oximetry in the neonatal intensive care unit (NICU): detection of hyperoxemia and false alarm rates. *Anesth Analg.* 2002; 94:S41–S43.

45. Ramsing T, Rosenberg J. Pulse oximetry in severe anaemia. *Intensive Care Med.* 1992;18:125–126.

46. Severinghaus JW, Koh SO. Effect of anemia on pulse oximeter accuracy at low saturation. *J Clin Monit.* 1990;6:85–88.

47. Severinghaus JW, Naifeh KH. Accuracy of response of six pulse oximeters to profound hypoxia. *Anesthesiology.* 1987;67:551–558.

48. Palve H. Comparison of reflection and transmission pulse oximetry after open-heart surgery. *Crit Care Med.* 1992;20:48–51.

49. Palve H, Vuori A. Pulse oximetry during low cardiac output and hypothermia states immediately after open heart surgery. *Crit Care Med.* 1989;17:66–69.

50. Rosenberg J, Pedersen MH. Nasal pulse oximetry overestimates oxygen saturation. *Anaesthesia.* 1990; 45:1070–1071.

51. Tittle M, Flynn MB. Correlation of pulse oximetry and co-oximetry. *Dimens Crit Care Nurs.* 1997;16:88–95.

52. Trivedi NS, Ghouri AF, Shah NK, Lai E, Barker SJ. Effects of motion, ambient light, and hypoperfusion on pulse oximeter function. *J Clin Anesth.* 1997;9: 179–183.

53. Chan MM, Chan MM, Chan ED. What is the effect of fingernail polish on pulse oximetry? *Am J Respir Crit Care Med.* 2003;123:2163–2164.

54. Cote CJ, Goldstein EA, Fuchsman WH, Hoaglin DC. The effect of nail polish on pulse oximetry. *Anesth Analg.* 1988;67:683–686.

55. Kataria BK, Lampkins R. Nail polish does not affect pulse oximeter saturation. *Anesth Analg.* 1986;65:824.

56. Ralston AC, Webb RK, Runciman WB. Potential errors in pulse oximetry. I. Pulse oximeter evaluation. *Anaesthesia.* 1991;46:202–206.

57. Ralston AC, Webb RK, Runciman WB. Potential errors in pulse oximetry. III: Effects of interferences, dyes, dys haemo globins and other pigments. *Anaesthesia.* 1991;46:291–295.

58. Rubin AS. Nail polish color can affect pulse oximeter saturation. *Anesthesiology.* 1988;68:825.

59. Scheller MS, Unger RJ, Kelner MJ. Effects of intravenously administered dyes on pulse oximetry readings. *Anesthesiology.* 1986;65:550–552.

60. Sidi A, Paulus DA, Rush W, Gravenstein N, Davis RF. Methylene blue and indocyanine green artifactually lower pulse oximetry readings of oxygen saturation. Studies in dogs. *J Clin Monit.* 1987;3:249–256.

61. Amar D, Neidzwski J, Wald A, Finck AD. Fluorescent light interferes with pulse oximetry. *J Clin Monit.* 1989; 5:135–136.

62. Block FE Jr. Interference in a pulse oximeter from a fiberoptic light source. *J Clin Monit.* 1987;3:210–211.

63. Brooks TD, Paulus DA, Winkle WE. Infrared heat lamps interfere with pulse oximeters. *Anesth.* 1984;61:630.

64. Fluck RR Jr, Schroeder C, Frani G, Kropf B, Engbretson B. Does ambient light affect the accuracy of pulse oximetry? *Respir Care.* 2003;48:677–680.

65. Siegel MN, Gravenstein N. Preventing ambient light from affecting pulse oximetry. *Anesthesiology.* 1987;67:280.

66. Fiechter FK. Results of a quality assurance study on the use of pulse oximetry in the postanesthesia care unit. *J Post Anesth Nurs.* 1991;6:342–346.

67. Gabrielczyk MR, Buist RJ. Pulse oximetry and postoperative hypothermia. An evaluation of the Nellcor N-100 in a cardiac surgical intensive care unit. *Anaesthesia.* 1988;43:402–404.

68. Van de LA, Cracco C, Cerf C, et al. Accuracy of pulse oximetry in the intensive care unit. *Intensive Care Med.* 2001;27:1606–1613.

69. Kelleher JF. Pulse oximetry. *J Clin Monit.* 1989;5:37–62.

70. Severinghaus JW. History and recent developments in pulse oximetry. *Scand J Clin Lab Invest.* 1993; 214:105–111 (suppl).

71. Tremper KK, Barker SJ. Pulse oximetry. *Anesthesiology.* 1989;70:98–108.

72. Bashein G, Syrory G. Burns associated with pulse oximetry during magnetic resonance imaging. *Anesth.* 1991;75:382–383.

73. Miyasaka K, Ohata J. Burn, erosion, and "sun"tan with the use of pulse oximetry in infants. *Anesthesiology.* 1987;67:1008–1009.

74. Murphy KG, Secunda JA, Rockoff MA. Severe burns from a pulse oximeter. *Anesthesiology.* 1990;73:350–352.

75. Rubin MM, Ford HC, Sadoff RS. Digital injury from a pulse oximeter probe. *J Oral Maxillofac Surg.* 1991; 49:301–302.

76. Wille J, Braams R, van Haren WH, van der Werken WC. Pulse oximeter-induced digital injury: frequency rate and possible causative factors. *Crit Care Med.* 2000;28:3555–3557.

77. Attin M, Cardin S, Dee V, et al. An educational project to improve knowledge related to pulse oximetry. *Am J Crit Care.* 2002;11:529–534.

78. Bilgin H, Kutlay O, Cevheroglu D, Korfali G. Knowledge about pulse oximetry among residents and nurses. *Eur J Anaesthesiol.* 2000;17:650–651.

79. Pedersen T, Pedersen P, Moller AM. *Pulse oximetry for perioperative monitoring.* Cochrane. Database. Syst. 2001; Rev.CD002013.

80. Keogh BF. When pulse oximetry monitoring of the critically ill is not enough. *Anesth Analg.* 2002;94: S96–S99.

81. Rutherford KA. Principles and application of oximetry. *Crit Care Nurs Clin North Am.* 1989;1:649–657.

82. Schnapp LM, Cohen NH. Pulse oximetry. Uses and abuses. *Am J Respir Crit Care Med.* 1990;98:1244–1250.